Understanding/Responding

A Communication Manual

for Nurses

Second Edition

Lynette Long, Ph.D.
Licensed Psychologist

Jones and Bartlett Publishers
Boston

Editorial, Sales, and Customer Service Offices
Jones and Bartlett Publishers
20 Park Plaza
Boston, MA 02116

Library of Congress Cataloging-in-Publication Data
Long, Lynette.
    Understanding/responding : a communication manual for nurses / Lynette Long. -- 2nd ed.
        p.   cm.
    Includes bibliographical references and index.
    ISBN 0-86720-433-8
    1. Nursing--Psychological aspects. 2. Communication in nursing.
3. Nurse and patient.   4. Interpersonal communication.   I. Title.
    (DNLM: 1. Communication--nurses' instruction. 2. Interpersonal Relations--nurses' instruction. 3. Nurse-Patient Relations. WY87 L848u)
    RT86.L66   1992
    610.73' 069' 9--dc20
    DNLM/DLC   91-35347
    for Library of Congress   CIP

Cover: Hannus Design Associates. Photo by David Powers/Stock, Boston   **173774**

Photo Credits
Page 1, Stock, Boston/Cary Wolinsky; page 13, Stock, Boston/ Rhoda Sidney; page 29, Stock, Boston/David Powers; page 39, Stock, Boston/Hazel Hankin; page 47, Stock, Boston/Jim Harrison; page 127, Stock, Boston/Cathy Cheney; page 187, Stock, Boston/Fredrik D. Bodin; page 227, The Picture Cube/ William Thompson; page 269, Stock, Boston/Paul Fortin; page 319, courtesy of George Mason University/Carl Zitzman.

Printed in the United States of America
95 94 93 92 91   10 9 8 7 6 5 4 3 2 1

*This book is dedicated
to my two wonderful children,
Seth and Sarah.*

Contents

Preface

The first edition of *Understanding/Responding: A Communication Manual for Nurses* was awarded "Book of the Year" by the American Journal of Nursing. The reviewers claimed, "This book should be quite useful to students who are learning to talk to patients, as well as to the seasoned nurse who needs a refresher in the always difficult area of communication."

The text is unique in its focus on nurses as delivery agents and its in-depth focus on the verbal and nonverbal communication of both empathy and respect. Through didactic material, programmed exercises, and simulation activities, the text presents the knowledge and skills necessary for successful nurse-patient interaction. The text is the result of more than twenty years of experience in teaching human relations. The excercises and activities in the text were field tested on approximately 1000 students, who successfully achieved the goal better interpersonal communications.

The exercises in the text are presented in a series of branched programs. Careful attention to the analyses of both the correct and incorrect responses will provide the reader with a greater understanding of the subtleties of interpersonal communication. The structured interviews provide the reader with an opportunity to view the entire process and the simulation activities provide practice in listening and responding to real-life situations.

The second edition of *Understanding/Responding* adds a new dimension to an already successful textbook. A new chapter on questioning has been added, which teaches students how to use questions effectively. Through a combination of didactic material, programmed excercises, and simulation activities, students learn when to ask a question, how to phrase facilitative questions, and when questions are

counterproductive. A second chapter containing five structured interviews has also been added. These interviews give
the reader an opportunity to view an entire conversation between a nurse and four different communication situations:
young children, an angry patient, a relative, and a dying patient. All in all, the text offers nurses a more complete training experience.

Lynette Long
Bethesda, Maryland

Understanding/Responding
A Communication Manual
for Nurses

1
Communication

The Heart of
Humanistic Learning

Nursing as a Relationship
Facilitating Components of Communication for
*   Building Relationships*
Nurse-Patient Relationship
The Manual: A Means of Integrating the Science
*   and the Art of Nursing*
Helpful Hints

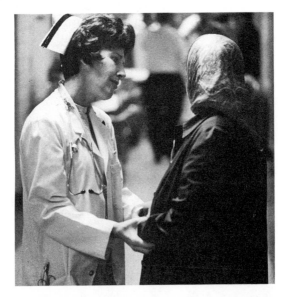

NURSING AS A RELATIONSHIP

Nursing is a dialogue— a human-to-human event. It's an experience that involves a meeting of human beings. No matter what theory of nursing is espoused, all that is nursing involves the process of human-to-human relating.

The means for attaining the goals of nursing through communication and relationship building are the main concern of this manual. The concepts that form the bases for communication and, ultimately, for building relationships are attending, listening, perception, caring, disclosure, acceptance, empathy, authenticity, and respect. Questions that are frequently asked by beginning nurses who are learning interactional skills are "How do these components of interpersonal dialogue relate logically and sequentially?" and "Which component must come first?" It is tempting to assign one factor as the crucial element necessary to initiate the understanding/responding process. But all of the elements of communication are closely interrelated. You cannot practice acceptance, for example, without also practicing a certain amount of disclosure as well. Empathy, respect, and genuineness have been identified as basic factors in the facilitation of relationships (Carkhuff & Berenson 1967; Truax & Carkhuff 1967), but one also could suggest that attending is a necessary precondition for realizing these elements (Egan 1985).

There will always be a certain circularity in any attempt to distinguish a "first" in the communication process. Each person possesses in varying degrees the necessary components of the communication dynamic. Rather than individual parts inserted into the interaction, however, the components are intertwined in the communication process with varying emphasis and timing. The goal of the understanding/responding process for humanistic nurses is not to "solve" people as you would solve a problem but to explore the mystery that is another person. From such an exploration you can learn about others and about yourself at the same time. Although you can never learn all there is to know about another person, human dialogue is in itself integrating and healing. A powerful moment in the dynamic of communication that makes possible a deeper experience of the relational nature of nursing is the moment when there is simultaneous understanding between nurse and patient.

Communication is the basis of humanistic nursing. To understand and communicate requires respect and a belief in the significance, worth uniqueness, goodness, and strength of the other person and in his or her capacity for and right to self-direction. Nursing is more, however, than a benevolent, technically competent rendering of services. It is also a responsible, caring relationship, and the meaningfulness of this relationship demands thought that is founded on awareness of yourself and the self of the other person.

Communication requires understanding of another's internal frame of reference, and this understanding can enable the two people involved to transcend their role relationship and establish authentic dialogue. True communication is capable of profoundly influencing and effecting community in its fullest sense. It is through communication that the uniqueness of the individual can be revealed.

FACILITATING COMPONENTS OF COMMUNICATION FOR BUILDING RELATIONSHIPS

Communication has many components: presence, listening, perception, caring, disclosure, acceptance, empathy, authenticity, and respect.

Presence, or attending to another, means seeing him or her in a very broad sense. The true meaning of attention is not anticipation, but acceptance and interest. Presence, however, cannot be achieved instantaneously; it requires time to develop.

To *listen* is to be open to the words, thoughts, and feelings of the other, whether these are expressed or implied. Listening requires sensitivity, understanding, and the withholding of any judgment of the other; it does not include taking responsibility for or attempting to mold the other person. Listening is an active, conscious effort to be present, rather than a mere passive reception. It requires a great deal of concentration, an open mind, and an interest in what is being said, in addition to the mere understanding of the meaning of the words spoken. To be a good listener, you must focus complete attention on the other, and this requires that your own prejudices, biases, preoccupations, and any other internal or external distractions be suppressed. For the nurse, listening facilitates recognition of the patient's needs, whether they are expressed verbally or nonverbally. The nurse who is an effective listener not only hears what the patient is saying but also looks for recurring "themes" in the patient's words.

Communication is based on respect for the other's *perceptions*. Actions are a direct result of one's perceptions, or frame of reference, so understanding another involves understanding that person's point of view.

Caring for another involves helping the other to grow and to actualize the self. In order for a caring relationship to exist, Mayeroff (1972) suggests that knowing, patience, honesty, genuineness, trust, hope, and courage must be communicated. Caring for another involves extending yourself. Caring is an essential component of nursing practice. For a nurse to care is more than "to take care of"; it is "caring for" and "caring about" as well.

Disclosure is the process by which the self is revealed to another; it is the reciprocal, dyadic process necessary for the development of a healthy personality (Jourard 1971). Thus, self-disclosure is essential for self-actualization. Because it is fundamental for self-knowledge and growth, self-disclosure is a necessary precondition for communication and for the implementation of various curative processes in therapeutic relationships.

Rogers (1965,1972,1983) has consistently noted that if one offers a person a relationship marked by respect, congruence, and the *acceptance* of feelings, the person will grow quite naturally toward healthy becoming, maturity, and responsibility. To accept another is to help him or her grow. Acceptance is akin to forgiveness: you weigh the behavior of the other and acknowledge the undesirable or negative aspects of that behavior, but you intentionally deemphasize these aspects while at the same time bringing into sharper focus those characteristics that are most pleasing and reassuring to the other. In accepting the other person, you do not impose directions for growth; rather, you allow the direction of the other's growth to guide what is communicated and to help determine how you respond and what is relevant to such a response. It is as if, by accepting the patient, the nurse allows the patient to accept himself or herself.

The ability to perceive the internal frame of reference of another with accuracy has been defined by Truax and Wargo (1966) as *empathy*. Empathy may be likened to putting yourself in the place of the other so that you see the other as he or she does. The empathic nurse mirrors and is present to the patient. Such a nurse is attuned to the present thoughts and feelings of the patient and verbally and nonverbally conveys this understanding. There is not only attentive listening to every word spoken and sensitivity to overt verbal expressions of thoughts and feelings but also a continual assessment and clarification of the meaning behind the communication. Empathy is crucial for the establishment of a facilitative interpersonal relationship, and it is also essential for the promotion of self-initiated experiential learning as well. In an atmosphere of understanding, the patient is freer to rediscover self, to grow, and to find new meanings that may be more accurate and more positive.

Authenticity is a prerequisite for a trusting relationship. Authenticity, or genuineness, means that a person is honest in sharing thoughts, feelings, and experiences with another. There is no artificial facade; when a person is what he or she appears to be, communication is said to be congruent. The authentic, or congruent, person is one who is aware of internal feelings and thoughts and who expresses these accurately, both verbally and nonverbally. This congruency is essential to meaningful communication. It promotes and sustains self-trust as well as trust between self and other. This trust gradually elicits uninhibited and open communication.

Rogers (1965) has described *respect*, or positive regard, as the perception of being positively valued. Respect conveys warmth, liking, and acceptance. According to Patterson (1985), respect involves the acceptance of another as a person of worth; it communicates a deep caring for another person despite that person's weaknesses. Interest in the development of the other person and belief in that person's ability to solve problems and choose positive actions are both a part of respect. Positive regard for another can be even more powerful than self-regard, and the experience of being respected as a person is essential for health and growth.

The components of communication provide the climate and the nourishment for understanding. They are the basis of listening and responding.

NURSE-PATIENT RELATIONSHIP

The responsibilities of a nurse are broad and complex. In order to be effective, nurses must exhibit two distinct areas of competence. First, nurses must demonstrate the cognitive and technical abilities necessary to the medical component of their work. In this area, qualified nurses are medically current and competent, have a thorough understanding of physiological functioning, have assessment and decision-making skills sufficient to insure the adequate care of the patient, and exhibit the technical skills to implement the patient's treatment plan. Second, nurses must have the behavior competencies necessary to interact with the patient in a therapeutic manner. In this role, nurses provide caring, comfort, instruction, and therapeutic listening.

Functioning in this domain as a "psychologist" or "crisis intervention specialist," nurses respond to the psychological needs of a unique and demanding group of patients. Their tasks are further complicated by the variety of roles in which they function, the extensive amount of time they spend with their patients, the sensitive nature of the content of the interactions, the lack of choice in selecting patients, and the imbalance of power between nurse and patient. These five areas each provide a challenge to the listening and responding skills of nurses.

The variety of roles in which nurses function. When interacting with patients, other health professionals, including doctors, physical therapists, X-ray technicians, respiratory therapists, and lab technicians, all interact with patients in a clearly defined role. Contrast these health professionals with nurses who fulfill a myriad of roles and a variety of functions in a patient's treatment. Nurses coordinate the patient's treatment, assess the patient's health and response to treatment, care for the patient's bodily hygiene, fill the patient's dietary needs, keep medical records, administer medication, take and record vital signs, conduct routine medical procedures, and serve as a liaison between the doctor, patient, and other health professionals.

In addition, nurses, are expected to listen to the patient. She is the patient's friend, counselor, and advisor; but at other times she is expected to administer procedures that are painful, say no to patient requests, or deny a patient attention because at that time another patient is more needy. These other nursing roles inhibit rather than foster her role as the "therapeutic partner" in the patient's care.

The extensive amount of time nurses and patients spend together. Hospitalized patients may spend 10 minutes a day meeting with their physician, from 30 to 60 minutes with a physical therapist, and limited and random contact with an X-ray or laboratory technician. Nurses, on the other hand, work an eight-hour shift in which they are either in direct contact with the patient or within close physical proximity to the patient. Depending on the patient's needs, the nurse will have numerous contacts with the patient on a daily or even hourly basis. This frequent and extended contact makes the nurse-patient relationship more intense than the patient's relationship with other health professionals.

This extended contact places a tremendous strain on the nurse. "Never off stage," she does not get much needed psychological rest. Psychologists, consummate professional listeners, only see patients for one hour at a clearly defined time in a clearly defined role and setting. They are not expected to slip into their role as a professional listener without warning—the way nurses are often required to do. If a psychologist sees a patient one hour a week, it will take two months before he or she has the same amount of potential contact with a patient as a nurse does on a single shift.

The sensitive content of nurse-patient interactions Nurses discuss personal information with patients on a daily basis. It is not uncommon for nurses to talk to patients about their bodily functions, sexual behavior, fear of dying, weight, or a critical diagnosis. Nurses see patients at their most vulnerable moments, when they are scared, in pain, or naked. They know whether a patient has false teeth, wears a wig, or has a prosthesis.

Often, nurses are expected to talk to patients regarding sensitive topics when sufficient time has not elapsed to build a close relationship with the patient that would permit discussion of these topics naturally. Psychologists talk to patients about sensitive topics but the timing is different. When a patient reveals sensitive information to a psychologist, it is usually how and when the patient wants to, whereas a patient may be forced to reveal sensitive topics to a nurse on the first day of contact.

The lack of choice. Once admitted to the hospital and assigned to a floor, patients do not have a choice of the nurse assigned to care for them—nor do nurses have a choice of the patients placed under their care. In some sense, the nurse-patient relationship is a forced relationship, brought together by circumstance, not by choice.

Consequently, nurses may be expected to care for and build a relationship with patients with whom they have no natural rapport. The relationship between a psychologist and a patient is one of self-selection. If the patient does not like a psychologist, then the patient does not return. If a psychologist does not think he or she can work effectively with a patient, then the psychologist may end the relationship.

The imbalance of power in the nurse-patient relationship. Although it is commonly said that nurses and patients are partners in the care of the patient, the reality is that the nurse has a tremendous amount of power when compared to the patient. The nurse, a professional in the medical community, has access to information the patient does not have, and has knowledge and experience the patient cannot match. Consequently, when it comes to the care of the patient, the nurse, and other health professionals, and often the patient, give greater weight to the nurse's perceptions, judgments, and opinions. Adding to this imbalance, the nurse controls the flow of goods and services to the patient. For example, medication prescribed on an as-needed basis is controlled by the nurse.

This imbalance of power between a nurse and patient inhibits trust and openness. It's very likely that the patient may be thinking, "How can I tell you what I'm really thinking when you might tell my doctor that I don't like him," or "If I'm honest with you, you might get mad at me and then you wouldn't give me any more pain medication." Often, the patient finds himself or herself in a struggle to be honest with the nurse and yet try to please her, since the nurse controls so much of the patient's life. The nurse is the patient's access to information on a variety of goods and services, and many patients worry that offending the nurse will result in a denial of that access.

THE MANUAL: A MEANS FOR INTEGRATING THE SCIENCE AND THE ART OF NURSING

This manual provides a skills approach to helping. In light of initial research efforts in nursing that focus on components of the communication process (Kalisch 1971; Kratochvil 1969) and in light of the attempts that have been made to improve the ability of nurses to empathically communicate, a theory-guided practical approach to teaching the components of communication seems essential. Studies by Carkhuff (1969) demonstrate that educational programs can be used effectively to increase an individual's measured levels of empathy, genuineness, and respect in communication. Although Carkhuff's primary method involves the use of rating scales (see Carkhuff's Appendix for the Empathy, Genuineness, and Respect Scales), too much emphasis often is placed on the discrimination of responses at different levels and not enough emphasis is placed on the formulation of responses. Students using the rating-scale approach become accurate rater, but they rarely receive practice in forming responses.

This manual utilizes a unique strategy designed to provide nurses with the basic interpersonal-communication skills they need to express to patients the caring and concern they feel. Our aim is to instruct nurses in the theory-based communication skills that will enable them in their interactions with patients to (a) encourage self-disclosure, (b) increase self-worth, (c) promote a deeper level of understanding, (d) increase both parties' satisfaction with the interaction, and (e) encourage problem solving and appropriate decision making.

This manual teaches the nurse to be a facilitative, person-centered helper. As helper, the nurse assumes responsibility for communicating the fact that the speaker's words have been heard; the nurse as facilitative helper takes an active interest in the patient and is self-disclosing. The nurse cares about the patient and struggles for self-understanding as well as facilitating the patient's self-understanding. By setting general guidelines for facilitative helping in both verbal and nonverbal domains, the manual provides the theory base for practical decisions. By emphasizing a person-centered philosophy and a foundation of scientific skills, the manual encourages the professional nurse to blend science and art. Through the exercises, the nurse formulates decisions that reflect appreciation of the scientific component, the skills component, and the art of helping as they are used to increase self-knowledge and understanding. This blending of science, skills, and art (see Figure 1) can lead to more effective communication and greater understanding not only between nurse and patient but also between nurse and colleague and between the nurse and members of the patient's family.

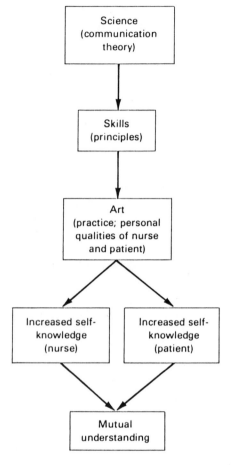

Figure 1. Integration of Science, Skills, and Art Leads to
Understanding

HELPFUL HINTS

This manual contains several kinds of materials. Key
concepts are explained, and programmed exercises are provided to illustrate the concepts in action and to help you
consider the implications of the various decisions in the exercises. It is best not to omit any of the exercises, because
much of the theory and many of the concepts presented in
the manual are developed within the context of these exercises. The sequence of the manual is cumulative, from basic
to complex.

Programmed materials are of two basic formats: branched and linear. The branched programs each present a problem situation and three possible responses. The response you choose determines the page you read next. It can be helpful, after completing a branched program, to go back and read all of the pages you were instructed to skip. These pages provide additional information about why particular responses are appropriate or inappropriate. The linear programs present you with a question, and you are to fill in the blank with an appropriate response. The desirable responses to these questions are located on the following page along with an explanation of why that response is appropriate. You will understand the concepts and your personal style of response best if you fill in the blanks before you consult the answer and explanation provided.

As you study the manual, try to practice the concepts presented. Watch the responses of other people as you practice your newly developed skills on them and try to learn from their responses to you. By integrating these skills into your normal communication patterns, you can become a more perceptive and effective professional.

Nurse/Patient Communication

Basic Concepts

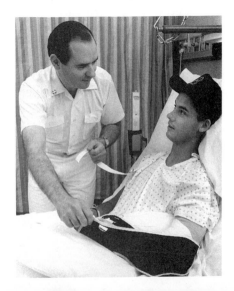

Consider the following dialogue between two nurses:

Brenda: Marge, I'm having problems communicating with a patient of mine who has cancer.

Marge: Oh, don't worry about it. Say, what's the date today?

Brenda: The 10th. He just lies there, and even when I try to open up communication with him after giving a pain medication or something, he doesn't respond.

Marge: Probably he just wants to rest. These new charts are awful! Where does the problem list go?

Brenda: Right here. There's the beginning work. I don't know what to do; I'm very worried about him. I want so badly to help him, because I can see that he's suffering and trying so hard to be brave.

Marge: Oh, it'll work out all right. He just doesn't want to talk.

At first glance you might find it difficult to believe that anyone could be as remote and insensitive to Brenda's concern as Marge appears to be. Yet, conversations like this surround us each day—conversations in which people are talking *at* each other but not *with* each other. These interactions happen everywhere: in homes, in crowded buses, in restaurants, and, of course, in health-care settings.

Everyone has the need to be listened to and understood. In most of us, this need is unsatisfied. We are seldom *heard* to our satisfaction; that is, we are seldom *understood.* People don't listen to us long enough, often enough, or well enough. Many of us feel unheard and thus unloved.

Often we share our thoughts and feelings in the hope that someone is listening but the knowledge that no one is. Brenda knew that Marge wasn't listening, but the situation with the suffering cancer patient was so disturbing to her that she preferred talking to Marge about it to keeping it to herself. Most of us find ourselves in this situation from time to time, needing to talk with someone else so much that we impose our conversation on people who really don't want to hear.

In searching for an appropriate listener, confidant, or friend, all of us test those around us. We share with each prospective listener a small piece of a problem or concern. Then we watch carefully to the response. Does the person seem interested? Does the person have the time to listen now? Is the person sympathetic? Will I be criticized? Will my problem be kept a secret? These are only a few of the many questions we ask ourselves before disclosing concerns to another.

PATTERNS OF INAPPROPRIATE RESPONSE

Patients ask themselves many of these same questions about nurses, and nurses respond in a variety of ways. Some communicate understanding and caring to their patients, and as a result share their concerns, fears, sufferings, and problems with the nurse. However, there is always the possibility of communicating one's lack of understanding and lack of interest in the patient's problems. This might be done in a number of ways. Here are a few of the more common responses that reflect poor listening, lack of respect, and lack of understanding.

Let Me Show You How Smart I Am.

This kind of nurse is more concerned with impressing the patient than with listening to the patient's problem. The nurse uses the patient's problem to demonstrate both her general knowledge and her problem-solving ability. She floods the patient with a barrage of information and solutions rather than demonstrate genuine caring and understanding.

Mr. Harris: I don't know what to do. I was taking a walk yesterday before I checked in here for these tests when suddenly my neighbor's dog ran up and bit me. It's not bad, really, but it did bleed for a while. I'm worried that it might cause me problems.

Ms. Cooper: I suggest that you tell your physician immediately. You'll need to have a tetanus shot, and then you have to decide whether you want to get rabies shots. The dog will have to be impounded. If it has been vaccinated for rabies and it shows no signs of rabies at the end of the impounding period, the shots will be unnecessary. Even if the dog is a carrier, however, you might not be one; even if you are, the helpfulness of the shots is questionable.

Let Me Tell You A Story.

This nurse listens long enough to get an idea of the problem and then begins to tell a story of her own. She is interested in the patient only as someone to listen to her, and she uses the patient's words only as a cue to share her own experiences.

Ms. Carson: Ms. Lillis, may I talk to you for a minute?

Ms. Lillis: Sure, what's up?

Ms. Carson: I slept poorly last night, and I really don't feel up to my treatment right now. May I take it later in the day?

Ms. Lillis: Why couldn't you sleep?

Ms. Carson: My Dean called last night at eight o'clock to tell me there was no one to take over the clinical practicum for my students. I felt guilty and worried about it all night.

Ms. Lillis: When I was an instructor a few years ago, I had to be admitted in the hospital unexpectedly for an appendectomy. The director of the school called me the next night and talked about how I should've prepared for that kind of emergency. She really gave it to me. It was hours before I could get some rest, and I began feeling much more pain and discomfort. They had to call the doctor in again in the middle of the night.

Not Now—Later.

This kind of nurse's response indicates no time for listening. The nurse postpones patient requests by minutes, hours, or even days. Often his postponement is actually an attempt to forget about the patient's request altogether. On the surface, the nurse seems concerned, telling the patient "I'm interested but not now." This type of response can be more destructive than the response of the obviously uninterested nurse.

Ms. Baker: Mr. Moran, may I talk to you for a minute, please?

Mr. Moran: I can't right now. This has been one of my busiest days.

Ms. Baker: But, Mr. Moran, it's important!

Mr. Moran: I'll talk to you after I chart my medications if you like. Why don't you take a nap right now?

Everything's Going to Be All Right.

This nurse doesn't take patient concerns seriously. She reassures patients with shallow statements such as "Cheer up," or "You'll feel better tomorrow," or "I know what you mean." She never really listens to or hears the patient's problem. She thinks she is being helpful, but because she never permits the patient to express himself or herself completely, the nurse "short-circuits" the helping process.

Mr. Jeffers: Ms. Constantine?

Ms. Constantine: Yes, what is it Leo?

Mr. Jeffers: I don't know really, I just don't feel right.

Ms. Constantine: You're probably just tried.

Mr. Jeffers: No, I've been sleeping at night and quite a bit during the day. Something's bothering me. I feel like nothing's worth doing.

Ms. Constantine: Don't worry. You'll snap out of it. You'll feel better about everything tomorrow.

Let's Talk about This Instead.

This kind of nurse indicates by his or her response a difficulty in listening to patient problems. Instead of admitting this to the patient and being authentic, however, the nurse changes the subject to something more pleasant. By constantly leading the patient away from the major concern at hand, the nurse ensures that the interaction will remain at a shallow level. Such responses indicate the nurse's fear of dealing with a serious patient problem.

Mr. Garcia: I'd like to talk to you a minute about something.

Ms. Flanders: Sure. What is it?

Mr. Garcia: It's my brother. Sometimes I get so mad at him I don't know what to do. This morning he called and said he'd taken my car keys and was going to use my car while I'm here in the hospital.

Ms. Flanders: What kind of car do you have?

Mr. Garcia: It's an old VW, but I've worked hard fixing it up. Anyway, when my brother told me he was taking the car, I lost my temper. We were both upset, and I said some awful things to him. Now I'm worried about him. When he's upset he often goes driving, and I'm afraid he'll hurt himself.

Ms. Flanders: I'd never go driving to calm down. Driving always makes me tense.

I Have the Answers.

This type of nurse tries hard to be helpful. The advice provided is not usually problem specific, but rather is based on a set of beliefs or ideas. Patients who interact with this type of nurse feel talked to rather then communicated with.

Mr. Golding: Mr. Lynch, could I talk with you?

Mr. Lynch: Yes. What can I do for you?

Mr. Golding: I don't know what to do. Nothing's getting better; I don't know whether to just leave the hospital or stay here and keep getting nowhere. They can't seem to find out what's wrong with me. All I can think about is the money this is costing and that I need to get back to work.

Mr. Lynch: If you leave the hospital on your own, you'll be sorry. Stick it out. You'll be glad in the end.

I'm Too Busy.

This kind of nurse is too busy to listen to the problems of patients. She is usually found checking I & O forms, looking over charts, filling out requisitions, checking monitors, and so forth. She does a fine job of communicating her preoccupation with hospital-related materials and equipment, and patients seldom ask for help. When they do, however, they're told that she's too busy.

Walt: Ms. Braun?

Ms. Braun: (Checking chart) Yes?

Walt: May I speak to you for a minute?

Ms. Braun: Not now; I have so many charts to check that it's going to take me quite a while.

Walt: Well, could you come to my room after you've finished?

Ms. Braun: By then it will be time for my report. I just can't today; I'm too busy.

I'm a Nurse, Not a Psychiatrist.

This kind of response indicates a perception of the nurse's role as that of technician and skilled caregiver. The nurse is willing to talk about health-related problems but fails to recognize the need of patients to express health-related psychological and personal concerns.

Ms. Stone: Mr. Shaw, could you help me?

Mr. Shaw: I'll try. What is it?

Ms. Stone: I'd like to talk to you about a problem I'm having.

Mr. Shaw: OK, go ahead.

Ms. Stone: Well, I was supposed to be discharged today, but now Dr. Winters has decided not to let me go because he thinks I'm depressed.

Mr. Shaw: Well, your doctor knows best. He'll probably call in a consulting physician or psychologist to help.

Ms. Stone: But what can I do about feeling so worthless and down?

Mr. Shaw: Why don't you wait and talk to your doctor and see if he can help you with your problem?

Here's What You Should Do.

This kind of nurse prematurely gives advice and provides solutions. He's ready to tell the patient what should be done without listening to the problem. The patient usually responds to the advice with "Yes, but ..." statements.

Patty: (Crying)

Mr. Davis: You're going to be all right, Patty. Don't cry.

Patty: But you don't understand. I...

Mr. Davis: (Interrupting) I understand just what you're feeling, and I think you should just tell yourself that you're going to get better. It always works. The only way to tackle this is to pull yourself together.

Patty: (Still sobbing) Yes, but ...

We're Always Cheerful.

This kind of nurse maintains a superficial attitude of cheerfulness that conveys an unauthentic concern for the patient and a lack of effort on the part of the nurse to be present to the patient and to share in understanding communication. This nurse uses cheerfulness to maintain distance.

Mr. Andrews: Ms. O'Brien, I've been wanting to talk with you about a problem I'm having.

Ms. O'Brien: Oh, I'm sure everything will work out OK.

Mr. Andrews: I just can't seem to...

Ms. O'Brien: (Interrupting) Let's take our bath now and we'll feel so much better. Won't that be nice? Why, look at those pretty flowers somebody brought you! They should cheer you up.

All of these nurses discourage further patient communication. Most do not do so intentionally, and some of them may even have thought they were being helpful. Most nurses sincerely care about their patients and would like to help when problems arise; however, many lack sufficient skills to comfortably and authentically communicate with patients— and with others—concerning personal problems. They don't know how to demonstrate the concern they feel and respond with understanding.

GOALS

This manual is designed to provide nurses with some basic communication skills that will help them to avoid the pitfalls illustrated by the sample dialogues above. Its aim is to teach nurses to be facilitative listeners in their dealings with patients. The facilitative listener cares about the person and what is being communicated and works to understand the person and to help the person to understand himself or herself.

KEY ELEMENTS IN COMMUNICATION

Communication is the medium for relationship building and involves both giving and receiving information. Two key elements of communication are the sender and the receiver. The person who gives the information is termed the *sender*, and the person who receives the information is the *receiver*. In the dialogue between Brenda and Marge at the beginning of this chapter, both women were senders and receivers. When Brenda spoke, she was the primary sender and Marge the primary receiver. (The term *primary* is employed because, even when Brenda is sending verbal messages to Marge, she is receiving nonverbal messages from Marge.) Thus, both Brenda and Marge are senders and receivers simultaneously.

The *message* itself—what is said as well as the corresponding nonverbal communication (attitude toward sender, message, and listener)—forms the third key element of communication. The words used, the body language, and the tone, inflection, loudness, and pitch of the voice are all parts of the message being sent. The fourth element is the response the receiver makes to the message, which is called *feedback*. The fifth key element is the *context*, or setting, in which the interaction occurs. Context is one of the most important elements involved in the meaning of the interaction. Each of the key elements is necessary for communication.

Because all five elements of the communication process reflect the experiences, thoughts, and feelings of the people involved, distortions or misunderstandings can occur. The content of the message is determined by what the sender thinks, feels, and perceives and by how he or she wants to be perceived by the other person. The receiver's perception of the message is structured by his or her perception of the world, which, in turn, is based on the receiver's perception of self within the context of the message received. In addition, the message and the feedback both are subject to distortion because of the limitations of language.

GENERAL GUIDELINES FOR LISTENING/ UNDERSTANDING

A few general guidelines for effective listening should be explored before we deal with specific facilitative-listening skills. You are probably familiar with many of these "rules" even though you've never verbalized them. These guidelines are intended to help you think about your listening behavior and to help you listen to others in the most facilitative manner possible.

Stop talking.   It seems almost ridiculous to say it, but in any conversation only one person can talk at a time. The easiest way to encourage disclosure is to provide the other person with an opportunity for disclosure by talking less yourself. Decreasing the focus on yourself increases the focus on the patient. Don't interrupt with questions or comments; instead, give the patient a chance to say all that he or she wants to say.

Get rid of distractions.   A good listener focuses completely on the speaker. This is easier to do if the environment is free of distractions. Ringing telephones, interruptions by other people, and noises from machinery or equipment can be distracting. In addition, it is difficult to talk to someone who is reading a newspaper, tapping a pencil, looking out the window, playing with a rubber band, or flipping a paper clip. Don't be guilty of allowing outside distractions to interfere with a conversation if this can be avoided, and never allow yourself to cause a distraction. Give the speaker your full attention.

Look at the speaker   Let the patient know that you are interested in what is being said. Sit in a relaxed and open position facing the patient, and don't be afraid to have eye contact. Looking at the patient will not only help the patient to communicate with you, but also help you to better understand the communication. This does not mean that you should stare but that you should be fully attentive and present.

Listen for the main point.   Listen for a theme or repeated idea in the communication. Concentrate on this theme and not on the details that embellish it. Ask yourself "What is this person trying to tell me?"

Listen to how the message is given.   Concentrate not only on what is said but also on how it is said. Listen for and be sensitive to emotional responses and attitudes. Ask yourself "How does this person feel about this situation?"

Separate the person from the idea. Often individuals are more influenced by who is saying something than by what is being said. We react more positively to the ideas of people we like than we do to the ideas of people we dislike or are indifferent to. It is difficult to separate the person from the idea, but try to listen very closely to patients you have strong feelings toward and be cautious of your interpretations. Listen to these people as though they were someone else. This will help you to hear more accurately what the individual is saying.

Listen for what is avoided. You can learn much about another person by listening for what is not said. Ask yourself "Has this patient omitted a significant part of the story? Does she avoid talking about her feelings or about a significant person in her life?"

Let the patient direct the conversation. The patient should determine the direction and the flow of the communication. By following his or her lead, you will more likely get to the heart of the matter quickly. You can be most helpful by letting the patient explore his or her own thoughts. It is the telling that is important for the patient. It is listening to the conversation, not directing it, that is central to the role of the nurse.

Be patient, don't interrupt. Allow the patient plenty of time to speak. After the patient stops talking, wait three seconds before you respond. This three seconds of "wait time" gives the patient sufficient time to complete a sentence or add a new thought.

Don't criticize. Criticism is the quickest way to put a patient on the defensive and make him or her stop the conversation. One critical comment can substantially reduce the patient's trust in you, which will take hours or days to rebuild. Criticism is highly destructive. If you are naturally critical, think before you speak.

Listen to the patient's feelings. Understanding a patient's feelings is central to understanding the patient. If feelings are expressed, be sure to paraphrase them. If feelings are implied, state what was implied. Never ignore a person's feelings.

Tell the patient how to reach you. Patients don't only need to talk when you are there. Explain how you can be reached when needed, perhaps saying, "Use the call light to reach me."

Explain to the patient when you are off duty. Often a patient will wait for a certain nurse, unaware that she got off duty at 11:00 or that today's her day off. Tell your patients, "I'll be here until 3:00." When you leave, tell your patient when to expect to see you: "I'm leaving now and tomorrow is my day off. I'll see you on Friday."

Separate you emotions from your responses. A difficult challenge but a crucial skill for a facilitative listener is the ability to separate emotional response from listening and understanding. Avoid the strong emotions of anger and sadness that may prevent you from hearing accurately and from responding with understanding.

Be careful with interpretations. Making hasty assumptions or jumping to conclusions can be dangerous. Assumptions are usually based on your knowledge of yourself, rather than your knowledge of the speaker. Don't assume that the speaker always uses words the same way you do, has the same values you have, or suffers the same weaknesses. Avoid interpreting the speaker's words and actions in light of yourself. Listen for facts, and be sure you know the difference between what was actually said and your interpretations, evaluations, or extrapolations of the facts.

Respect the patient as a person. There must be genuine respect, interest, and caring for and about the other person if you are to be really helpful. You must value the patient and all his or her communications and take the time and make the effort to listen.

Empathize with the person. Empathy is often defined as putting yourself in the other person's place so that you can see the world as that person does. The empathic listener offers understanding, not solutions, and tries sincerely to understand the person as he or she is and to perceive the other's frame of reference.

Patient Requests

In the nurse-patient relationship, there is a difficult balance of power. Because nurses have access to information that the patient does not and because nurses control the supply of goods, services, and information to the patient, they have tremendous power in their relationship with the patient. On the other hand, nurses fulfill a service function for the patient; in essence they are employed by the patient to care for him or her. When the patient emphasizes this service function of the nurse by making a request, the balance of power shifts.

To a patient, there is no such thing as a trivial request. Sometimes the patient who only asks for a glass of water or a magazine is actually asking for reassurance. He or she is really saying, "I don't want to be alone. Can you sit and talk for a minute?" or "I'm scared. What's going to happen to me next?" Instead of making themselves vulnerable, many patients express their fears and concerns indirectly. Listen clearly for the underlying message.

Honoring a simple request is a good way to build a relationship with a patient. When you get a patient a glass of water, the patient often thinks, "She's nice," or "She cares." Later, when a crisis occurs and the patient needs to talk to someone, the patient will often trust the nurse who took the time to show she cared.

If a patient overwhelms you with requests, don't get angry or say no. Rather, help the patient prioritize his or her requests. A simple statement like, "I can't do everything you asked right away. What's most important to you?" will help reduce the stress of multiple requests and still leave the patient feeling heard.

If you can't honor a patient's request, say so at the time. Don't respond by saying, "I'll see" or "Maybe" when you really should say no. It is better to deny the request and explain the reason for your refusal. Patients often make requests that conflict with their treatment or that discourage independence. Patients can accept an answer of no when they understand the reason why. Vague responses will only build up a patient's hopes and cause problems later.

TALKING TO PATIENTS

Nurses don't only *listen* to patients; they *talk* to them. To the nurse, the hospital is a place of employment; it holds no mysteries. But to a patient, a hospital is an alien environment, often frightening and confusing. Nurses are usually the patient's most accurate and frequent source of information. Accurate information diminishes fear and helps the patient cooperate more fully with treatment.

Recognizing that their doctor is busy and sometimes feeling intimidated by him or her, patients generally refrain from asking the doctor too many questions. Instead, the patient expects the nurse to outline the treatment plan, work out the daily schedule, clarify the function and doses of various medications, explain routine and not-so-routine procedures, and inform the patient of hospital rules and regulations. Keeping the patient will-informed is a time-consuming and often difficult task, especially since patients differ in their desire for information, the intensity with which they pursue it, and their ability to understand it. Here are a few pointers that can help you in your role as a teacher.

Explain procedures to the patient.   Take the time to explain what is going to happen next. Don't let a patient worry about something when a few minutes of your time can relieve days of anxiety. Routine procedures that are performed dozens of times a day in any hospital are foreign to the patient. Patients may worry that an EKG or sonogram will hurt. Although it seems preposterous to you, it only proves that most patients don't know what to expect. Many experts caution that too much information heightens fear. To the contrary—information *reduces* fear.

Avoid jargon.   Medical jargon and abbreviations only make procedures seem more frightening and complex. Professionals often use initials to describe procedures because they are efficient and represent a common base of knowledge. But patients don't know what these initials stand for and it only makes them feel more helpless and frightened. Use complete words when explaining procedures to a patient and define medical terms in everyday language.

Take the time to answer questions thoroughly.   When a patient asks a question about his or her treatment plan, answer the question thoroughly. Don't just give a one-sentence answer to the question. Go through the entire procedure step by step and use clear language and nonmedical terms.

Anticipate questions.   Many patients have difficulty asking questions. They may sit and worry about tomorrow's CAT scan without asking a single question about the procedure. Prepare the patient by explaining the entire procedure. Don't lead with, "Tomorrow you're going to have a CAT scan—do you know what that is?" The patient will more than likely respond, "Yes" because he or she does not want to appear stupid. Instead, start with, "Tomorrow you're going to have a CAT scan. Let me tell you a little about it." Once you start, it's up to the patient to interrupt if he or she doesn't want to hear your explanation. Even patients who had a procedure explained to them earlier may find a second explanation reassuring.

Assume the patient knows nothing.   The most effective teachers assume the student knows nothing. The nurse, often functioning as the patient's teacher, should also assume the patient knows nothing. Assume the patient has never before been in a hospital and is unfamiliar with even routine procedures such as an IV.

Don't respond to "What if?" questions with technical information.   "What if" questions often signal deeper patient concerns rather than a need for technical information. For example, a patient who asks, "What if the cancer spreads to my bones?" or "What if my baby is deformed?" is not asking for technical information but rather is voicing fears. Instead of responding to the technical question asked, respond to the hidden fear: "You're afraid your cancer is spreading," or "You're worried that your baby may be deformed." Technical answers such as, "If you have bone cancer, your doctor will probably prescribe radiation therapy," or "If your baby is deformed, the doctor will order a variety of tests to determine the nature of the deformity so that an appropriate treatment plan can be developed," will only heighten the patient's fears and ignore the need for reassurance.

The following chapters provide a detailed methodology for effective understanding and responding. With practice and time, these skills can become a part of your unique and personalized approach to your patients.

3
Active Listening
in Problem Solving

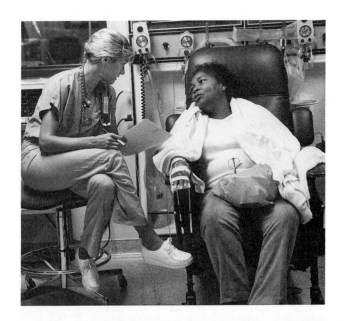

Ms. Lewis is upset and frustrated because her lab tests have been inconclusive. Mr. Herman is uncertain and frightened about the insecurities of retirement. Ms. Lyons is terrified when she learns that she has cancer of the lung. These and numerous other problems are likely to be presented to the nurse during any day at a hospital or clinic. When you hear such expressions of frustration, hurt, disappointment, and fear, you must decide whether to become involved with the patient in working through the problem. If you decide to do so, you must make known your willingness to become involved and be accepted by the patient as a potential helper. These steps set the stage for cooperative problem solving, growth, and change.

Setting the stage, however, does not mean solving the problem. Many nurses respond when their patients approach them with problems, but their responses often fail to facilitate constructive change because the nurses fail to follow some simple but crucial rules for understanding and responding. These rules are particularly effective when working with short-term situational problems.

There are some key stages in the problem-solving process. They are:

1. Disclosure, which includes both the expression of the problem by the patient and the expression of understanding and feedback by the nurse;
2. Problem definition, or consideration of all aspects of the problem;
3. Goal setting, or development of courses of action;
4. Goal evaluation, which follows the action that has been taken to achieve the goal.

These stages are generally sequential and will be discussed in the order given. Each stage is important for problem resolution(see Figure 2).

DISCLOSURE

In the first stage, disclosure, the patient's problem is presented in very broad terms. The patient might reveal the problem little by little or blurt it out in an incoherent, explosive, or rambling way. Sometimes the person is testing during the disclosure process to determine how safe it is to relate

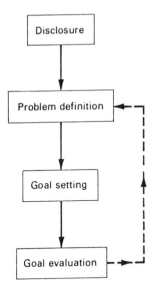

Figure 2. The Problem-Solving Process of Helping

authentically and to share his or her real concerns with the nurse; at other times the frustration of the unresolved problem has built up to such an extent that the patient is unable to contain the problem any longer and it bursts forth all at once.

The responses of the nurse during this stage are very important, because they let the patient know that it is safe to share thoughts and feelings and that the nurse is willing to hear the patient out. Initial responses should also communicate the nurse's understanding that there are many aspects to any problem and the nurse's assurance that she or he will not try to brush the problem aside with simple solutions. During disclosure the nurse should try to understand and to establish a relationship with the patient. Building this relationship involves developing in the patient a sense of confidence that the interaction will produce positive results.

During disclosure, listening is the nurse's most important activity. It allows the nurse to find a stable position from which to understand the problem and communicates to the patient the nurse's willingness to understand. Listening lets the patient know that, for the nurse, understanding is more important than generating an immediate solution. Listening by being present to the patient with warmth and genuineness facilitates the establishment of a relationship in which constructive change and growth can take place.

What do we listen for?   There are three major areas that the nurse should be most attentive to in this first stage:

1. The patient's description of the events that led up to the problem,
2. The patient's narration of his or her thoughts regarding the problem,
3. The patient's description of all the feelings he or she has had regarding the problem.

All three of these areas play an important part in understanding. The patient's thoughts and feelings about the problem are as crucial, if not more so, as the "facts" of the problem. People frequently are distressed not so much by the situations they find themselves in as by the view they take of those situations.

How do we encourage self-expression?   During disclosure the listener has three particularly helpful tools for encouraging the patient to elaborate on the problem and the thoughts and feelings that accompany it. These tools are the reflective response, the clarification response, and the summarizing response. If sensitively incorporated as part of the helping process, each can facilitate disclosure and deeper understanding.

The *reflective* response is the most basic of the three and is essentially a restatement or paraphrasing of the patient's significant disclosures. It says to the patient: "I have heard what you've said thus far,""I understand," and "It's OK to share your problem with me; I'm listening." Because the reflective response is a nonjudgmental one, trust is facilitated when reflective responses are used authentically. The nurse communicates that she or he is accepting the problem and not judging it or the patient. The reflective response is the most powerful means for encouraging patient disclosure.

Clarification responses state both the expressed and the implied content and feeling of the patient's disclosure. They say to the person: "I heard what you said, and I understand what you're feeling. I even understand some of the things you're afraid to say. Talk more deeply to me about this topic." The clarification response can prompt significant speaker disclosure that leads to greater understanding of the patient's frame of reference.

PROBLEM DEFINITION

The disclosure stage allows the establishment of the problem from the patient's point of view and provides a reciprocal exchange for the building of an interpersonal relationship. Once the patient has revealed the problem and the emotions and thoughts surrounding it, it's time to examine the problem in detail.

In this second stage it is important for the patient and the nurse to achieve a conscious understanding of all the details of the problem. Clarification is important in outlining the problem, defining perceptions, and determining reality. At this point the nurse should listen carefully to his or her own internal responses. When the thoughts and feelings the patient expresses differ from the thoughts and feelings of the listener, the nurse should try to clarify these differing perceptions. Often these internal responses provide helpful clues about which part of the problem needs further exploration and where disparities exist. This open exploration of the problem for conscious understanding leads logically to the task of defining all parts of the problem.

When patients present problems, they often are seeking not solutions but understanding. In the definition process the patient and the nurse work together to achieve a clear, realistic, and total picture of the problem, and the nurse can be particularly helpful by facilitating the patient's consideration of all aspects of the problem. It is sometimes difficult to get a clear picture of a situation in which one is deeply involved. The nurse, who is not directly involved in the problem, can provide the patient with a new perspective and might be able to detect aspects of the problem that are not apparent to the patient. The nurse also may be better able to discern which aspects of the patient's problem are pertinent and which are not.

Several kinds of responses are useful to the facilitative listener in this phase. Reflection communicates the listener's understanding of the patient's definition of the problem; this response acts as a mirror, helping the listener verify his or her perceptions. Clarification delineates aspects of the problem or highlights issues that may have been unclear; this response helps determine the extent of the problem and often elicits additional aspects of the problem that the patient finds difficult to explore. Questioning by the nurse can lead the patient to clarify the problem by filling in gaps in information. This ensures that all relevant data are presented.

A common mistake made during this stage of helping is the nurse's attempt to solve the problem for the patient. Both the nurse and patient may be tempted to have the nurse resolve the problem, but this should be avoided. In order for constructive and enduring change and growth to occur, the resolution of the problem must be generated and accomplished by the patient.

GOAL SETTING

Once the problem is clearly and completely defined, both the patient and the nurse should be ready to face the question "What can be done to resolve the situation?" This third stage begins when the nurse and the patient are unable to uncover any new information about the problem. When nothing more can be said to define the problem, the time for goal setting has arrived.

The purpose of the third stage of problem solving is to consider as many solutions to the problem as possible. The patient and nurse should work together to arrive at ways of resolving the problem. The major function of the nurse/listener at this point is to facilitate goal identification and goal setting by the patient. The nurse encourages the patient to generate solutions by asking questions such as "Can you think of any other solution?" and "How else might you handle this situation?" The nurse should support the patient's suggested solution by making statements that demonstrate understanding and awareness of the goal-setting efforts. Whether the nurse uses supportive statements such as "That's one good idea" or reflects the goals identified by the patient, both the patient and the nurse should feel that they are working together to arrive at possible solutions.

It's often difficult for people to see their way clear of problems in which they are deeply involved. A patient who has defined his or her problem may see only one solution, and this solution may be an unacceptable one. The patient may even see the problem as one with no solution—as a "hopeless" or "impossible" situation. At these times the nurse, who is hearing the problem for the first time and is not bound by the same psychological barriers as the patient, can be of great help. The nurse can be facilitative by thinking of possible goals or solutions that are not apparent to the patient. By this time the nurse should understand the problem almost as well as the patient, and no solution is too trivial or foolish to be considered. Even if the solution is without merit in itself, it might lead to another, more workable, solution. Any goals suggested by the nurse, of course, should always be presented as possibilities to be considered and not as prescriptions to be followed. Be careful, however, not to overwhelm the patient with your solutions.

The responses that are appropriate during the goal-setting stage include reflection, to communicate the listener's understanding of the solution suggested by the patient; clarification, to expand on the patient's solutions; and questioning, to clarify points or to elicit needed information and alternative solutions. At the end of the third phase, the patient and the nurse should feel that they have arrived at a number of possible solutions from which a final selection of the most appropriate goal or solution can be made.

GOAL EVALUATION

During the fourth stage the patient and nurse continue to work together to consider the advantages and disadvantages of each proposed solution or goal. The focus is not on thinking of ways out of the problem but on evaluating the solutions considered earlier. The nurse should help the patient to consider the consequences of each of the proposed solutions. Questions such as "What would happen if . . ." or "Can you think of any reasons why this wouldn't work?" might prove helpful. The pros and cons of each goal should be carefully outlined and weighed. After considering the advantages and disadvantages, the patient should feel that he or she is in a position to make a decision. The decision may not be easy, but the patient should feel that the decision is coming from a thorough exploration of the situation, an understanding of his or her own thoughts and feelings, and a thorough evaluation of the possible alternatives. When the final decision is made, it is the patient's alone to make; he or she alone will experience the consequences of that decision.

By encouraging the patient to make his or her own decision, the nurse encourages the patient to take responsibility for himself or herself and for the manner which his or her life is conducted. The nurse must not be critical of the patient's selection of a solution. Rather, the nurse should continue to support the patient no matter what path is selected. An effective listener will have communicated this acceptance to the patient during the decision-making process so that the patient feels free to make whatever choices he or she thinks is best. The nurse's comment at this stage might be "I've tried to assist you in exploring your situation. We've considered a number of possible alternatives, and now its up to you to decide what you want to do. I'll stick by you no matter what decision you make."

The process of evaluating solutions is facilitated by a number of different responses. Reflection is used to communicate an understanding of the patient's thoughts and feelings about the alternatives; clarification is used to help the patient to further explore the consequences of alternative solutions as well as explore his or her feelings about the alternatives. Questioning, although used to clarify statements, is probably more often used to seek relevant information and possible solutions from the patient.

Near the end of the goal-evaluation phase, both nurse and patient should have a feeling of accomplishment. They should feel that they've arrived at a solution to the problem and that this solution is based on careful consideration of all relevant aspects to the situation. The patient should feel that the decision reached represents his or her best efforts, given the circumstances. The patient should feel (1) that he or she has been understood and accepted by the nurse and (2) that the relationship is comfortable enough so that, if the situation is not resolved after the plan is enacted, the patient can return for continuation of the problem-solving process. The nurse, of course, should feel a sense of satisfaction in having helped another person.

You may find that you are tempted to rush through the first and second phases of problem solving in order to reach stages three and four. A listener often feels that the time spent on self-expression and problem definition is too slow and in some sense wasted, but that something is being accomplished when solutions are being generated and evaluated. Workable and satisfying solutions, however, are not likely to be based on superficial and hasty considerations or on vague outlines of the problem. The first two stages of problem solving should not be treated lightly, because time spent in these activities provides the foundation for the best resolution of the problem. All four stages are rarely completed in a single conversation; several sessions may be required so that both persons have time to closely consider the problem.

In summary, the problem-solving model comprises four *sequential* stages for the resolution of short-term problems, although in actual problem-solving situations there may be some overlap of these phases. The first stage, disclosure, and the second stage, problem definition, are likely to overlap, as are the stages of goal setting and goal evaluation. Some stages may even have to be repeated before a final decision is reached. While considering and evaluating alternatives, for example, a redefinition of the problem may occur, necessitating a return to stage two and progression again through stages three and four. Frequently, too, the process of self-disclosure aided by listener clarification will resolve the problem. Therefore, it should be stressed that the four-stage model presented in this chapter is intended as a guideline and not a rigid pattern to be followed inflexibly.

4
Nonverbal Methods for Facilitating Communication

Nonverbal Behavior
Structuring the Environment
Physical Cues
Vocal Cues

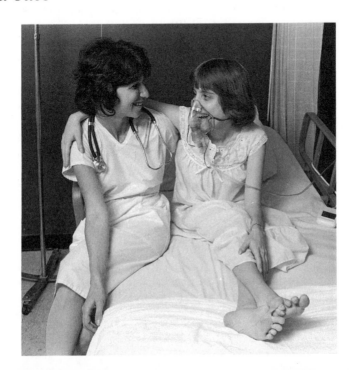

NONVERBAL BEHAVIOR

Nonverbal behavior encompasses all physical methods of communication except speech; it is what we do with our heads, eyes, hands, and legs. Nonverbal behavior permits the nurse to respond to the patient in an understanding, accepting, and caring way. That part of our communication that others see, rather than hear, is nonverbal. Nodding your head, slumping in your seat, clenching your fists, putting your hand on someone's arm, wringing your hands, breathing heavily, and perspiring profusely are all forms of nonverbal behavior.

Verbal communication is selective; we choose to speak or to remain silent. Nonverbal communication is constant. We are continuously sending physical messages that reflect our psychological and emotional state, even when we are sleeping. Nonverbal communication is eloquent for those who are sensitive to it.

Nonverbal behavior also differs from verbal behavior in the level of conscious awareness it requires of the sender. Speech is a conscious phenomenon. We are always aware of what we are saying, because the formulation of speech is an intellectual process that is always consciously controlled. What we say is not always a true reflection of what we think and feel, but it is symbolic of what we want to communicate about ourselves. Nonverbal communication is not always conscious; rather, it shifts in and out of our conscious awareness. Certain individuals, such as actors and politicians, have learned to be acutely aware of their nonverbal communication and to control it. But, for most of us, nonverbal behavior is usually an accurate representation of what we are thinking and feeling because we do not control it. Sometimes, in fact, the nonverbal message is so strong that it completely overrides the words the person is speaking. We don't control our nonverbal behavior very well. When we do become aware of this behavior, we're not always sure how to use it to communicate what we wish to say. Because of this general lack of control over nonverbal communication, it is frequently granted more validity then verbal behavior.

Nonverbal behavior is continuously being transmitted and continuously being received and interpreted by others. If our nonverbal communication is consistent with our verbal communication, it enhances our words and adds credence to them. But if nonverbal behavior and verbal behavior give conflicting messages, the receiver will frequently give greater weight to the nonverbal behavior because it is less likely to be masked or controlled.

The aim of this chapter is to increase your awareness of the role of nonverbal behavior in communication. It will provide you with guidelines for making your nonverbal messages more consistent with your verbal efforts to communicate respect and understanding.

STRUCTURING THE ENVIRONMENT

One of the first steps in communicating concern and interest to a patient and facilitating openness is the selection of an appropriate time and place to talk. The right environment will increase the likelihood of sharing, as well as the ease with which the patient discloses. Study the following guidelines and try to select a place in your working environment that meets these requirements.

Privacy

Privacy greatly enhances the likelihood of both relationship building and successful helping. A patient is not going to feel free to discuss a problem of any magnitude when there are others to overhear. Fear of losing control or appearing foolish in front of others will interfere with honest and open communication, even with the most willing patient. Pressing the patient for disclosure when you are in a public area or when other people are in the patient's room will prove unsuccessful. It will only communicate to the patient that you are insensitive to the need for privacy and the importance of the problem. It is better to wait until a private place can be found than to require a patient to discuss a serious problem in an environment that impedes open communication.

Freedom from External Distractions

After you find a private place to talk, you must make it relatively free from distractions. A classroom, lounge, or private room is fine as long as you won't be interrupted by other people. An office is even better, if the phone isn't ringing every five minutes. Remember that work also is a distraction. A nurse who sits behind a desk looking at all the charts to be written or constantly looking at the clock is distracting to the patient. Distractions interfere with the helping process in two ways. First, they interrupt the interaction; when conversation resumes, it will take time to recapture the train of thought and to return to the previous level of patient disclosure. Second, distractions communicate a lack of respect and lack of presence on the part of the nurse. They say to the patient "These interruptions are more important than our conversation."

Silence

Another key to a facilitative environment is quiet. Constant noise may or may not be distracting, but it usually is counterproductive. The constant rhythm of respirators, suction machines, and other equipment can provide constant background noise. Making oneself heard above these noises can be a definite stumbling block to open communication, because no one wants to shout out personal information. In fact, the most personal statements are usually spoken very quietly. If background noise is present, the nurse can easily miss an important comment by the patient. Asking to have the comment repeated often results in the response "Oh, nothing."

Spatial Arrangements

The arrangement of the room also affects the process of helping. Smaller rooms generally are better than larger ones, because they provide a sense of safety. Chairs, too, are important, because sitting down to conduct a conversation communicates to the patient that the dialogue will be more than a momentary one. It says "I have time to listen now" and communicates respect for the patient. The chairs should be soft and comfortable and placed directly facing each other. Spatial distancing and maintaining the patient's personal space are particularly important, so the chairs should be placed four to six feet apart. This is close enough to create a sense of intimacy but not so close as to be threatening to the patient. There should be no physical barriers such as desks, tables, other chairs, or hospital equipment between the nurse and the patient, because these can impede disclosure.

If the patient is confined to bed, lower the bed to a level at which eye contact can be maintained comfortably.

PHYSICAL CUES

Once the proper physical environment is provided, the nurse must see to it that his or her nonverbal responses, or physical cues, are consistent with the verbal communication taking place. Both the verbal and nonverbal messages must reflect respect and understanding. To achieve congruent verbal and nonverbal behavior, you must first be aware of the physical cues that most directly communicate respect and understanding and facilitate self-disclosure. Here are a few guidelines to consider.

Eye Contact

Maintaining eye contact is a key factor in facilitating nurse/patient communication and disclosure. Looking directly at a patient says "I am more interested in you than in the other things going on around us." It indicates a sincere attempt to understand the patient and also suggests "Talk to me; I'm listening." Eye contact should be established often enough and long enough to be encouraging but should not be so persistent that it makes the patient uncomfortable. Eye contact not only will facilitate disclosure but also will help you to understand the patient better (for example, a person's eyes will dilate when he or she thinks of pleasurable experiences).

Facial Expressions

The patient will be very aware of your facial expressions if you are maintaining regular eye contact. Because all of us use facial cues in forming impressions of others, these cues should be consistent with the emotions being expressed in the conversation. When the patient is animated, you should express interest; when the patient is sad, you should show concern; when the patient is happy, you should share that happiness through your expression. A nurse's facial expressions that conflict with the patient expressions of emotion are counterproductive. A nurse who is smiling when a patient is crying or looking sad when a patient is joyful is communicating a lack of understanding. Such obvious insensitivity will very probably end the interaction.

The nurse's facial expressions should be consistent not only with the patient's verbal and nonverbal expressions but also with the nurse's own verbal expressions. You should not be scowling while saying "I feel happy for you" or smiling when saying "You have a serious decision to make here." The key is to be natural and to give conscious consideration to your facial expressions only when they seem inconsistent with other communications. If your facial expression is inappropriate, you probably are experiencing some conflict; something that the patient is saying is triggering a strong reaction in you. If you see that your response is disturbing the patient, acknowledge that you're aware of your inappropriate response by saying something like "I know I'm smiling while you're obviously upset, but it's not because I don't feel your pain. I really don't know what's going on with me right now."

Body Posture and Position

Body posture also should be used to communicate understanding and respect. A good rule to follow when you are genuinely interested is to lean forward and tilt your head toward the patient. This communicates interest. Don't sit in a forced or rigid position; shift your position naturally. Try to convey to the patient not only that you are interested in what is being said but also that you understand. Nod appropriately. Your body movements and posture can encourage the patient and let him or her know that you are attending to the conversation.

Use your body to communicate interest and openness. Face the patient squarely. Do not sit at an angle, if possible. When you sit facing the patient, you're communicating interest and respect by saying "I'm serious about this conversation; my primary focus is you." Show openness to the patient's ideas by sitting in a relaxed and open position. Avoid crossing your arms or legs since this may be interpreted as an indication of closed-mindedness. Try not to hunch over or look tense; relax. Nonverbally communicate to the patient "I feel ready to accept whatever you're going to say. I'm approachable. Talk with me."

Touching

Touching can be a very meaningful nonverbal behavior. Because touch is one of the primary modes of communication, it is an important factor in nurse/patient interactions. The most basic way to make contact with another person is by touch; words can become unnecessary. Some form of physical contact with the patient can help to create the mutual openness that is necessary for the formation of a relationship.

Touching can bring the patient back to the conversation, facilitate verbal expression, relax the patient, provide comfort, or communicate that the nurse is there and understands. Touching can even express different meanings at different times; the same action, such as putting your hand on the patient's arm, can convey warmth, reduce anxiety, or communicate interest. Touching can be a powerful physical expression of a relationship.

VOCAL CUES

Vocal cues also are important in the nurse/patient interaction. These vocal cues are not *what* we say but *how* we say it. They can either reinforce or diminish the significance of our verbal and nonverbal communications.

Voice Rate

Voice rate is a key factor in communication. To communicate empathy, the nurse's voice rate must be somewhat consistent with the patient's speech pattern. A nurse who responds to a very animated patient comment by speaking very slowly communicates lack of understanding and lack of interest. Shifts in voice rate, although necessary, should be moderate. A response that is expressed too hurriedly could suggest to the patient that the nurse is feeling impatient. Speech that is too rapid communicates lack of respect; it says "I don't have time to listen to you now." On the other hand, speech that is too slow could imply boredom or lack of interest. Thus, to maximize the communication of understanding and respect, your voice rate should be varied to match the patient's expressed emotions but should never be so fast as to communicate impatience or so slow as to indicate boredom.

Voice Tone

Your tone of voice should be regulated in much the same way as your voice rate. It should vary according to what the patient is communicating but should never be extreme.

In summary, understanding is communicated non-verbally by behavior that is congruent with the feelings being expressed. Nonverbal behavior communicates "I am with you. I'm feeling what you're feeling. I am here for you and I mirror your thoughts and feelings." Respect is communicated non-verbally by behavior that is open and attentive and says "I have time to listen to all that you wish to share with me. I'm interested in your world. I care." When you find yourself not interested in the patient, or not valuing the patient as a person, question the situation. Perhaps the patient is not being honest and your lack of interest is a response to the lack of genuineness. If such discrepancies arise, it is wise for the nurse to take special note of them because they may well point to aspects of his or her own life that have not been adequately resolved. Struggle to understand your own inconsistent communications; the challenge can well result in growth for you. Read extensively in the area of self-awareness and self-development (for example, Watson & Tharp 1977; Jourard 1971). If it is difficult for you to communicate respect for a particular patient, ask yourself whether it is something in the patient that is triggering your reaction. Again, try to understand your reaction because this may provide helpful insights for you, which in turn will strengthen your ability to communicate with others.

5
Reflective
Listening

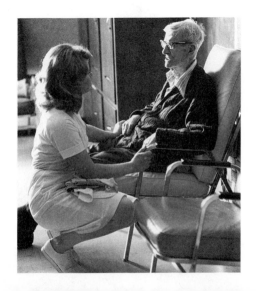

The first skill necessary for effective responding is listening. Most people not only don't hear much of what is said to them but also hear things that are not said. When asked to repeat the content of a message, they usually leave out one or several of the main points and often add content of their own.

A nurse's ability to repeat a message word for word is of little use to the patient or the nurse, but the ability to hear the message accurately and remember it is essential. A nurse who knows how to listen can choose which part of the message he or she is going to focus on in responding. A nurse who hears or remembers only part of the message, however, has a limited choice of responses. In fact, the nurse may have missed or forgotten the most essential part of the message. It's best to try to remember the whole message in the patient's own words, if possible.

Nurses who frequently add content to the patient messages they hear are not listening effectively. They are not focusing their attention exclusively on the patient; rather, while the patient is talking, their focus is on their own thoughts and feelings. These become entwined with the patient's message, resulting in the nurse's inaccurate recollection of the conversation. Try to focus your attention exclusively on the patient. Listening and understanding are hard work and require lots of practice and disciplined effort. The following exercises will help you develop these skills.

Listening: Exercise 1

A 62-year-old patient, Florence Greene, makes the following statement to the staff nurse as he walks into Florence's room.

> *Florence:* *I've been ringing this call bell for 20 minutes and no one has bothered to answer. What are you running here, a hospital or a social club for nurses?*

Try to remember, without looking back, exactly what Florence said to the nurse. Write your answers below.

Now look back and check the accuracy of your memory.

_____ 1. Did you remember Florence's statement word for word?
_____ 2. There were three main points in this patient's message. Did you recall all of them?
_____ 3. Did you only recall one or two of the main points?
_____ 4. Did you add any new content to the original message?

Listening: Exercise 2

The nurse walks in to check on Diane York, a 24-year-old patient. Diane is staring at the ceiling. After much prodding by the nurse, she makes the following statement.

> **Diane:** *I'm going to die. I just know it. I'm going to die. My whole life's over. And it hasn't even begun. It hasn't even begun!*

Try to remember, without looking back, exactly what Diane said. Write your answer below.

Now look back and check the accuracy of your memory.

_____ 1. Did you remember Diane's statement word for word?
_____ 2. Diane repeated two sentences for special emphasis. Did you repeat those two sentences?
_____ 3. Diane's statement contained four main ideas. How many did you remember?
_____ 4. Did you add any new content to Diane's original message?

Listening: Exercise 3

A 17-year-old patient, Robert Jackson, makes the following statement to the floor nurse when she asks him how he is feeling.

> *Robert:*   *I feel great! I get to go home tomorrow. With hard work, my leg should be as good as new in about six months. I'll even be able to play football again next season. My coach is really relieved!*

Try to remember what Robert said. He made five major points. List them below.

Now look back and check the accuracy of your memory. In this example, each major idea is contained in a separate sentence.

_____ 1. How many of the major ideas did you remember?

_____ 2. Did you add any new ideas to the original message?

Listening: Exercise 4

The staff nurse enters the room to administer routine medication to a 38-year-old patient, Richard Wilson. He greets the nurse with the following statement.

> *Richard:*   *Listen, nurse, I want the truth from you. I ask everyone who comes in here what's wrong with me and they all beat around the bush. One nurse says "What do you think is wrong?" and another tells me "Just be patient. Wait until the doctor arrives." Well, I'm tired of being patient! I have a family to support. What's wrong with me?*

Try to remember what Richard said to the nurse. He made eight major points. List them below.

Now look back and check the accuracy of your memory.

_____ 1. Of the eight main ideas in Richard's message, how many did you remember?
_____ 2. Did you add any new content to the original message?

If you remembered six or fewer of the ideas, you need more practice in listening. Work out a personal plan to practice and improve your listening skills.

THE BASIC REFLECTIVE RESPONSE

There are several ways to be a facilitative listener. The most simple of these is *reflection*. A reflective response accurately paraphrases the essence of the message. Such a response focuses on the patient and what he or she is trying to communicate. By repeating the essential parts of the message in only slightly different words, the nurse lets the patient know that he or she has been accurately heard. Notice that such a response is free from the nurse's own biases and value judgments because no new content is added.

If a patient, Karl, says to the nurse on duty, Mr. Barnes:

You know that nurse on the afternoon shift—the one with the red hair? She seems so incompetent. I don't like her at all.

An accurate paraphrasing of this message would be:

So, you think Ms. Aaron is incompetent, and you don't like her.

Karl feels that he has been listened to. He doesn't know whether Mr. Barnes agrees or disagrees with him, but he does know that the nurse has heard his opinion. He is now free to express why Ms. Aaron does not measure up to his expectations.

Compare Mr. Barnes' response, which summarizes the content of Karl's statement, with these other common nurse responses:

Nurse Response 1:   Ms. Aaron is a fine nurse. You have no right to be critical of her.

Nurse Response 2:   She doesn't have to be likeable—just competent.

Both of these responses reflect the values of the nurse. In the first response, the nurse evaluates both Karl and Ms. Aaron. In the second response, the nurse cites his own opinion on the essential qualities of nursing. In neither case does he show any understanding of how Karl is perceiving the situation.

The reflective response is the basis for all facilitative communication. It is absolutely essential in initial interactions with a patient. When a patient brings a problem or concern to a nurse, he or she may be testing that nurse's sensitivity to others. If the nurse responds in a way that communicates listening and understanding, the patient will probably continue to disclose relevant information. The patient's initial statement is usually only a superficial representation of the real problem. Only after the patient has tested the nurse's reaction will he or she disclose the more significant aspects of the problem. One way to initiate a climate of trust is to correctly use the reflective response. This response communicates "I hear and respect your feelings; trust me." Responding to a patient's initial statement with a response other than the reflective one can be risky; it's like trying to determine the picture on a jigsaw puzzle by using only one piece. Usually the game is stacked against you, because the patient often provides only a very unrevealing "first piece." Help the patient share his or her thoughts and feelings with you in more depth by using the reflective response.

Remember that, in responding to initial problem statements, reflection is almost universally the most helpful response. It is also one of the basic response styles employed in later nurse/patient communication.

Too often, nurses offer solutions to the problems patients present to them—solutions that the patient is usually aware of already. Most patients, when they present their problems, are seeking not solutions but understanding. You will notice that the reflective response does not offer solutions; rather, it demonstrates to the patient that the statement of the problem was heard as it was presented. Offering a patient quick solutions, instead of understanding and a willing ear, can often cut off communication.

Nurses may also reduce patient communication by making demands on the patient in the form of expectations. A nurse should never expect a patient to "live up to" the nurse's values. A reflective response helps the nurse avoid this kind of demand because it does not permit the nurse to communicate personal values. The reflective response contains no new information and does not add to or subtract from the patient's original statement.

Reflecting: Exercise 1

Reread the following statement by Robert Jackson. Which of the possible nurse responses is the most helpful?

> **Robert:** *I feel great! I get to go home tomorrow. With hard work, my leg should be as good as new in about six months. I'll even be able to play football again next season. My coach is really relieved!*
>
> **Nurse Responses:** A. *Don't be too eager to play football again. That leg of yours needs time to heal.*
> B. *I had a leg injury once. I was happy too when I found out my leg was going to be all right.*
> C. *You feel great because you get to go home tomorrow and because your leg will heal completely, allowing you to continue to play football.*

If you picked A, turn to page 60.
If you picked B, turn to page 61.
If you picked C, turn to page 62.

You picked A

> ***Don't be too eager to play football again. That leg of yours needs time to heal.***

This is not the most helpful response, because it gives the patient advice. It cautions him against playing football too soon and reinjuring the leg. This caution was not necessary, because Robert had already indicated that he knew how long it would take his leg to heal. His attitude did not reflect haste. Response A ignored Robert's good feelings and his happiness at his release from the hospital. It focused on only one of several issues mentioned by the patient. A reflective response would have been more helpful.

A reflective response is equal to the original message in content and feeling. It's an accurate paraphrase of the patient's statement, and it says "I heard what you said, and to prove it I'm going to repeat it back to you in my own words."

A response that reflected Robert's statement would repeat what he said in only slightly different words. It would include reference to his good feelings, his dismissal from the hospital, the healng of his leg, and the prospect of his playing football again.

Return to page 59 and pick out the reflective response.

You picked B

> *I had a leg injury once. I was happy too when I found out my leg was going to be all right.*

This is not the most helpful response. In this response the nurse discloses parallel information, which shifts the focus from the patient to the nurse. Her response focuses not on Robert's happiness but on her own past experience. It doesn't communicate interest in the patient and will probably discourage Robert from further sharing of his good feelings. Thus, Robert is robbed of an opportunity to completely experience his joy.

A reflective response would have been more helpful. It would focus on Robert and his message, not on the nurse. A reflective response, which is equal to the original message in content and feeling, is an accurate paraphrase of the patient's statement, showing the patient that the nurse heard what Robert said.

A response that reflected Robert's statement in only slightly different words would include reference to his good feelings, his dismissal from the hospital, the healing of his leg, and the prospect of his playing football again.

Return to page 59 and pick out the reflective response.

You picked C

> ***You feel great because you get to go home tomorrow and because your leg will heal completely, allowing you to continue to play football.***

Congratulations! This is the most helpful response—that is, a reflective response. It is equal in content and feeling to Robert's original statement. It tells him that the nurse heard what he said and shares his happiness, inviting him to talk further about his good feelings.

If you're not sure why the two responses you didn't choose were incorrect, go back and read the analyses of the other two responses. Then turn to page 63.

Reflecting: Exercise 2

A 38-year-old woman, Frances Williamson, made the following statement. Pick out the most helpful response the nurse could have made.

> *Frances: I'm scheduled for surgery tomorrow, but I don't want to go. I'm scared! Maybe I really don't need the surgery. Maybe I'll get better without it.*

> *Nurse Responses: A. What did your doctor tell you when he was in today?*
> *B. You're afraid to go to surgery tomorrow. You fear the operation might be too much for you.*
> *C. You wish you didn't need surgery and you hope that you'll get better without it. You're afraid to go to surgery tomorrow.*

If you picked A, turn to page 64.
If you picked B, turn to page 65.
If you picked C, turn to page 66.

You picked A

What did your doctor tell you when he was in today?

This is not the most helpful response. It poses an unnecessary question to the patient. It focuses not on Frances' present feelings of fear but on her previous conversation with the doctor. This response communicates a lack of understanding. Having Frances recall the earlier conversation would be of little value. She is already aware that the conversation took place, and it appears to be providing her with little comfort. This question might satisfy the nurse's curiosity and temporarily distract the patient, but it will provide little comfort and be of little lasting value.

A reflective response would prove more helpful because it would communicate an understanding of the patient's position. Reflective responses do not seek information; they allow the patient the privilege of deciding what information is to be shared. By repeating (reflecting) the original response, the nurse would encourage Frances to disclose more fully, secure in the knowledge that the nurse understood her original communication.

A reflective response would simply repeat the main ideas of Frances' original statements, focusing on her last-minute fear of surgery, her desire to avoid it, and her wish that she would get better without it.

Go back one page and try again.

You picked B

You're afraid to go to surgery tomorrow. You fear the operation might be too much for you.

This is not the most helpful response. It *interprets* the patient's original response. The nurse infers from Frances' statement that she fears the surgery might be too much for her—that she might die. Although this hypothesis might be correct, the nurse should not be the one to voice this concern. She should wait for Frances to continue her dialogue and state her fears herself. A response such as this one, touching the patient's innermost fears, can be very threatening to the patient at this time. Indeed, if the nurse's interpretation is incorrect, it will communicate a lack of understanding. In either case, such a response is not helpful.

A more helpful response would be a reflective one. This would communicate the nurse's understanding of the feelings Frances was expressing. It would not magnify the intensity of those feelings, as her interpretation does. A reflective response—repeating the original message—encourages the patient to disclose more fully because it communicates this understanding.

A reflective response would repeat the main ideas of Frances' original response, focusing on her last-minute fear of surgery, her desire to avoid it, and her wish that she would get better without it.

Go back two pages and try again.

You picked C

> *You wish you didn't need surgery and hope that you'll get better without it. You're afraid to go to surgery tomorrow.*

Congratulations! This is the most helpful response. It is a reflective response, repeating the major ideas in Frances' statement. The response tells Frances that her fears were heard just as she expressed them. It doesn't ask unnecessary questions or magnify the patient's feelings. It focuses entirely on the patient and her specific message.

If you're not sure why the two other responses were incorrect, go back and read the analyses of those two responses. Then turn to page 67.

Another time to use a reflective response is when you disagree with what a patient has said. Using this kind of response lessens the possibility of an emotional conflict, which often arises simply because two people are trying to make themselves heard and neither is trying to listen. When you demonstrate that you've heard the other person, you reduce the emotion behind the conflicting ideas of patient and nurse. (This works very successfully with patients who have complaints about hospital procedures.) Only after you have demonstrated that you've heard the patient should you give your own opinion. However, you should never give an opinion on specific patient feelings—only on external matters.

For example, a patient might say to you:

I think this is the worst hospital in the city! I wish I'd gone to Winston General; they have a much better staff.

Even though you disagree with the patient, you should demonstrate listening by responding with something like the following:

You're not satisfied with this hospital. You think Winston General has a better staff.

Because the patient is speaking about a situation as well as internal feelings, you can conclude your statement with your own feelings about the hospital, if you choose to do so. When a patient expresses internal feelings, it is detrimental to the free flow of communication for the nurse to make a judgment of those feelings. The only possible judge of the validity of an internal feeling is the person experiencing it.

Reflecting: Exercise 3

Mrs. Adams, a 43-year-old patient, made the following complaint to the day nurse. Select the most helpful response the nurse could have made.

Mrs. Adams: *I want to change my room. I can't stand sharing a room with this woman. She's constantly watching TV, and I never get a chance to rest. She's so inconsiderate!*

Nurse Responses:
A. *Why don't you try talking to Ms. Edwards about the situation?*
B. *You feel that Ms. Edwards is being inconsiderate by constantly watching television. You'd like to change your room because the TV interferes with your rest.*
C. *It doesn't appear to me that Ms. Edwards watches television excessively.*

If you picked A, go to page 69.
If you picked B, go to page 70.
If you picked C, go to page 71.

You picked A

Why don't you try talking to Ms. Edwards about the situation?

This is not the most helpful response. It offers a possible solution to the problem presented, and at first glance it appears helpful. But a closer look highlights some obvious shortcomings. Mrs. Adams began her remarks by suggesting a solution: having her room changed. The nurse's response suggests an alternative solution, which communicates to Mrs. Adams that her solution either was not heard or was not acceptable. Recognition of the patient's complaint and proposed solution should precede any other action by the nurse. This nurse's response will inhibit the nurse/patient relationship, because he is suggesting a solution that is apparently unacceptable to Mrs. Adams. He thereby communicates a lack of understanding of her situation. This patient called for the nurse's assistance either because she feels unable to talk to Ms. Edwards about the problem or because she has already tried unsuccessfully to talk to her. Ignoring the patient's concerns the way this response does only magnifies the patient's emotions and intensifies the problem.

A reflective response would prove more helpful. It communicates understanding, not solutions. A reflective response is a repetition of the main points of the original message, focusing on the patient and what is bothering her. A response that reflects Mrs. Adams' statement would repeat what she said in slightly different words and would include reference to the TV problem, the effect it has on her, and her proposed solution to the problem.

Go back one page and pick out the most helpful response.

You picked B

> **You feel that Ms. Edwards is being inconsiderate by constantly watching television. You'd like to change your room because the TV interferes with your rest.**

Wonderful! This is the most helpful response. It is reflective—equal in content and feeling with Mrs. Adams' original statement. It neither defends Ms. Edwards nor offers a solution. The nurse merely repeated the patient's message in different words. This response tells the patient that her complaint was heard and understood. It gives her further opportunity to discuss her feelings with the nurse.

Read the analyses of the two incorrect responses and then turn to page 72.

You picked C

> **It doesn't appear to me that Ms. Edwards watches television excessively.**

This is not the most helpful response. It negates the patient's experience. It not only does not communicate understanding but also voices a contradictory opinion. This response says to the patient, "You're wrong. Ms. Edwards doesn't watch TV excessively." A confrontation of this kind will force the patient to defend her perceptions and will increase her feeling of irritation. It's important to remember that it doesn't *matter* whether Ms. Edwards watches the TV excessively. All that should matter to the nurse is how Mrs. Adams perceives the situation, because what she believes is reality for her.

A reflective response would prove more helpful in this situation. It would communicate understanding, rather than the nurse's opinion. A reflective response would repeat the main points of Mrs. Adams' message, focusing on the patient and what is bothering her.

A response that reflects Mrs. Adams' original statement would include reference to the television problem, the effect it has on her, and her proposed solution to the problem.

Go back three pages and pick out the most helpful response.

Reflecting: Exercise 4

Read the following statement by a patient named Carol. Try to rewrite the statement in your own words without changing the content or feeling of the message. Include in your response all the main points presented by the patient.

> **Carol:** *I feel fantastic! They finally diagnosed the "tumor" in my stomach as an ovarian cyst. It's not malignant, and I don't even have to have surgery. What a relief!*

Write your paraphrase of this statement below.

There are many ways to paraphrase Carol's statement. Two possible paraphrases are listed below.

1. You found out that you have an ovarian cyst. You feel relieved because it's not malignant and because you don't require surgery. You feel fantastic.
2. You feel both fantastic and relieved that you found out you have a benign ovarian cyst and don't require surgery.

Paraphrase 1 begins by focusing on the factual information the patient related. It deemphasizes Carol's feelings by responding to them in two separate parts of the message. Paraphrase 2 begins by focusing on Carol's present feelings. It responds to both feelings together, giving them added importance.

Reflecting: Exercise 5

Read the following statement by a patient named Arnie. Try to rewrite this statement in your own words without changing the content or feeling of the message. Try to include in your response all the main points presented by Arnie.

> **Arnie:**   **I came to this hospital to feel better, but nothing you do here seems to do any good. I still feel terrible, and I still don't know what's wrong with me. I wish I could just feel good for a change.**

Write your paraphrase of this statement below.

There are an unlimited number of ways to restate Arnie's message. Here are three of them.

1. You feel terrible. You wish you would just feel better. You expected hospital treatment to help, but you don't think it has. You don't know what's wrong with you.
2. You came to the hospital to feel better but so far have had no results. You still feel terrible. You don't know what's wrong but just wish you would feel better.
3. You don't know what's wrong with you. You still feel terrible. You came to the hospital for help, but nothing seems to work. You wish you would feel better.

Although essentially the same, these three responses differ slightly in their focus. Paraphrase 1 emphasizes the idea that the patient feels terrible. Paraphrase 2 emphasizes the lack of progress being made at the hospital. Paraphrase 3 emphasizes the confusion the patient is feeling. These differences are slight but do exist because of the order in which the ideas are presented in each paraphrase.

DISCRIMINATING BETWEEN EXPERIENCE, COGNITION, AND AFFECT

In responding to any statement by a patient, the nurse must decide to which aspect of the patient's communication she or he is going to respond. The nurse can respond to the experiential, the cognitive, or the affective component of the message or to any combination of these. The experiential component is that part dealing with the experience itself, the cognitive component is that part dealing with the patient's thoughts about that experience, and the affective component is that part of the message dealing with the patient's feelings about the experience.

The experiential component of the message is defined as the patient's account of incidents that happened to himself or herself or to others. The cognitive component of a message can include thoughts about something as concrete as an experience or about something as abstract as an idea. The feelings the patient expresses make up the affective component, which is purely emotional. Thus, a patient's message can contain as many as three component parts. The first answers the question *What happened?* The second answers the question *What does the patient think about what happened?* The third answers the question *How does the patient feel about what happened?*

Some messages will not have all three components. Messages such as "Boy, am I mad!" and "Do I feel great!" have only affective, or emotional, content. Statements such as "I had a pain pill two hours ago" and "I can't walk very far" are free of thoughts and feelings and are meant to express only observable events or experiences. Examples of purely cognitive statements would be "I think this room needs to be painted" and "I think he's feeling better today."

The nurse who reflects the patient's statement responds only to what is presented by the patient. If only an affective component is presented, the nurse must confine his or her response to that component. Similarly, if only a cognitive component is presented, the nurse must respond only to that cognitive material. No new material is added by the nurse in a reflective response. However, most messages contain at least two of the three components, so the nurse must decide whether she or he is going to respond to all or only to some of the components presented.

Here is an example of a message with all three component parts. Following it are seven possible combinations of the components to which the nurse could choose to respond.

Harvey: Every time I need to go to the bathroom, I have to ring this bell. Then one of you comes in to help me. I'm embarrassed. I don't know—I just think a man of my age should be able to handle those things himself.

1. The nurse could respond only to the experiential component:

    At your request, a nurse comes to help you when you need to go to the bathroom.

2. The nurse could respond only to the cognitive component:

    You think you should be able to go to the bathroom by yourself.

3. The nurse could reflect only the patient's affective statement:

    You feel embarrassed.

4. Reflections of combinations of these components are also acceptable. Reflecting all three components is easy:

    You have to call a nurse every time you need to go to the bathroom. You're embarrassed because you think you should be able to handle that yourself.

5. Another option is to respond to a combination of the affective and cognitive components:

    You're embarrassed because you think you should be able to go to the bathroom by yourself.

6. The nurse could choose to ignore the patient's feelings and respond only to the experiential and cognitive components:

    You think you should be able to go to the bathroom by yourself, yet you have to call a nurse.

7. Finally, the nurse could choose to ignore the cognitive component and respond only to the experiential and affective components:

    You feel embarrassed because you have to call for a nurse every time you need to go to the bathroom.

At its best, the reflective response contains the experiential, the cognitive, and the affective components of the original statement. Sometimes this is impossible, because all three components are not always represented in the original statement. When a patient's statement contains only a cognitive component, for example, the nurse can reflect only the cognitive component. When patients realize you're listening to their thoughts, however, they're more likely to trust you and reveal their feelings. Experiential and cognitive content are only as important to the patient as his or her feelings about that content. The statement "I had a pain pill two hours ago" is void of any emotional content and is not, in itself, meaningful for the nurse other than as simple information. What is important is how the patient feels about having had a pain pill two hours ago. Is she happy about it because it's still providing needed relief, is she irritated because there has been such a delay, or is she without any particular feelings about the pain pill? The original statement is a neutral one. Its only importance is in the impact that the experience related by the patient has on her. Feelings are always paramount to the speaker. Therefore, the nurse should always respond to any feelings that are being expressed. A good rule of thumb is to reflect the major experiential and cognitive components and to never ignore the affective component. Trivial details of the patient's actions in response to the experience may be ignored and the cognitive component can be condensed, but be sure to include the affective component in its entirety and in an intensity similar to that of the patient.

Most nurses think they can differentiate feelings from thoughts, but this is something few people have ever really learned. Sometimes patients use the expression "I feel" to introduce cognitive components: "I feel that Bill is a good doctor" or "I feel that I'll be better next week." Both of these statements could better be introduced by "I think" or "I judge that" or "I believe," because they contain thoughts, rather than feelings. Patients, like most of us, have probably found that feelings are taken more seriously than thoughts by most people, so they try to "sneak" their thoughts in under the label of feelings. At times all of us confuse our thoughts with our feelings, and at times we are simply afraid to express our feelings. Thus, what may appear to be affective disclosure is in reality no more than cognitive disclosure, which requires less trust. Interestingly enough, the reverse of this phenomenon seldom occurs. How often do you hear a patient say "I think mad" or "I think disappointed"?

In summary, there are three possible component parts of a message. Any message can have one, two, or all three of these.

1. What happened?
   a. This is the speaker's experience.
   b. It contains the description of an external event.
   c. The reported event may be an observable incident, written material, or the reported thoughts and feelings of another person.
   d. This is the experiential component of the message.
2. What does the patient think about what happened?
   a. These are the speaker's thoughts.
   b. They contain the speaker's cognitive, or mental, reaction to the experiential component.
   c. This is the cognitive component of the message.
3. How does the patient feel about what happened?
   a. These are the speaker's feelings.
   b. They contain all "gut-level" reactions, or emotional content.
   c. These may include the speaker's feeling about the experiential component and his or her feelings about the cognitive component.
   d. This is the affective component of the message.

Here is a breakdown of Florence Greene's message, which we encountered earlier.

> **Florence: I've been ringing this call bell for 20 minutes and no one has bothered to answer. What are you running here, a hospital or a social club for nurses?**

What happened? (experience):

> *I've been ringing this call bell for 20 minutes and no one has bothered to answer.*

What does the patient think about what happened? (cognitive reaction):

> *What are you running here, a hospital or a social club for nurses?*

How does the patient feel about what happened? (affective reaction):

> *(Although this patient's sarcasm indicates that she is obviously irritated, she doesn't express her anger directly.)*

Discriminating: Exercise 1

Read the following statement by a patient named Edna. Break it down into its three component parts.

> **Edna: *I'm so happy. My daughter came to visit me last night. She flew in all the way from Texas! She must really care about me.***

What happened? (experience):

What does the patient think about what happened? (cognitive reaction):

How does the patient feel about what happened? (affective reaction):

Here is the correct breakdown.

> **Edna: I'm so happy. My daughter came to visit me last
> night. She flew in all the way from Texas! She must
> really care about me.**

What happened? (experience):

> *My daughter came to visit me last night. She flew in all the
> way from Texas!*

What does the patient think about what happened? (cognitive
reaction):

> *She must really care about me.*

How does the patient feel about what happened? (affective reaction):

> *I'm so happy.*

Discriminating: Exercise 2

Read the following statement and break it down into its three component parts.

> ***Mrs. Steinberg:*** *My son's really sick. They want me to leave him here until the end of the week for tests. I don't know if I can live without him. I'm scared.*

What happened? (experience):

What does the patient think about what happened? (cognitive reaction):

How does the patient feel about what happened? (affective reaction):

Here is the correct breakdown.

> **Mrs. Steinberg: My son's really sick. They want me to leave him here until the end of the week for tests. I don't know if I can live without him. I'm scared.**

What happened? (experience):

My son's really sick. They want me to leave him here until the end of the week for tests.

What does the patient think about what happened? (cognitive reaction):

I don't know if I can live without him.

How does the patient feel about what happened? (affective reaction):

I'm scared.

Discriminating: Exercise 3

Read the following statement and break it down into its three component parts.

> **Mr. Underhill:** **I'm so mad at that doctor! He didn't show up this morning to sign my discharge papers.**

What happened? (experience):

What does the patient think about what happened? (cognitive reaction):

How does the patient feel about what happened? (affective reaction):

Here is the correct breakdown.

Mr. Underhill: I'm so mad at that doctor! He didn't show up this morning to sign my discharge papers.

What happened? (experience):

He [the doctor] didn't show up this morning to sign my discharge papers.

What does the patient think about what happened? (cognitive reaction):

(This is not stated.)

How does the patient feel about what happened? (affective reaction):

I'm so mad!

Discriminating: Exercise 4

Read the following statement and break it down into its three component parts.

> ***Janet:*** *I haven't had a visitor for days. Even my husband hasn't come to see me! I feel that you're the only person who cares what happens to me.*

What happened? (experience):

What does the patient think about what happened? (cognitive reaction):

How does the patient feel about what happened? (affective reaction):

Here is the correct breakdown.

> *Janet: I haven't had a visitor for days. Even my husband hasn't come to see me! I feel that you're the only person who cares what happens to me.*

What happened? (experience):

I haven't had a visitor for days. Even my husband hasn't come to see me!

What does the patient think about what happened? (cognitive reaction):

I feel that you're the only person who cares what happens to me.

What does the patient feel about what happened? (affective reaction):

(This is not stated.)

(Notice that, although this patient begins one of her sentences with the phrase "I feel," her thoughts—not her feelings—are being expressed.)

SELECTED REFLECTIVE RESPONSES

It's important for a nurse to be able to discriminate among a patient's experiences, thoughts, and feelings in order to respond in the most helpful manner. Previously, we indicated that the nurse has seven possible avenues of response in reflecting a patient's statement. However, if the patient's experiences and thoughts are considered one unit and are called the *content* of the message, the number of available responses is reduced to three. The nurse can now choose to respond (1) only to the content (experience and thoughts) of the patient's message, (2) only to the patient's feelings, or (3) to both the content and the feelings expressed in the patient's message. It's up to the nurse to consider the alternatives and reflect that part of the message that will best communicate his or her understanding of the patient's message. Examine the nurse's response to the following statement by a patient's husband.

Mr. Birchall: It's my wife—she's dying. I'm afraid to go in there and see her. I can't act cheerful, and it won't do her any good to see me upset.

1. *Nurse's Response (to the content of the statement):* You don't want your wife to see that you're upset because she's dying.
2. *Nurse's Response (to the speaker's feelings):* You're afraid.
3. *Nurse's Response (to both the content and feelings expressed by the speaker):* You're afraid of getting upset in front of your wife.

All three responses reflect different components of the speaker's message, but all three are not equally helpful. Response 3 is the most helpful. It communicates to Mr. Birchall that the nurse understands both how he feels and why he feels that way. Response 1 is less helpful because it ignores Mr. Birchall's feeling of fear, which is the most significant part of his communication. Response 2 is less helpful than response 3 because it does not communicate an understanding of why Mr. Birchall feels the way he does.

Generally, the most helpful response is one that reflects both the content and the feelings of the speaker's message. All feelings, of course, should always be reflected. Unfortunately, feelings are the least likely thing to be disclosed by the speaker and the most likely thing to be ignored by the listener. A facilitative listener encourages the expression of feelings by always responding to any feelings expressed. In contrast, it is not necessary to reflect all of the content contained in the message. The selective listener reflects only that content that is significantly related to the feelings expressed. The nurse should focus on the content that communicates to the speaker the nurse's understanding of why the speaker feels the way she or he does.

Selective Responding: Exercise 1

Read the following patient statement and decide which of the nurse responses is the most helpful.

> *Mr. Biener:*   *I feel great. We had a daughter! We already have two sons, Tom and Mike. We wanted a little girl more than anything. She's beautiful.*

> *Nurse Responses:*   A. *Your wife gave birth to a daughter.*
>   B. *You got your wish. You wanted a daughter because you already have two sons.*
>   C. *You feel wonderful. You got the daughter you wanted.*

If you picked A, turn to page 92.
If you picked B, turn to page 93.
If you picked C, turn to page 94.

You picked A

Your wife gave birth to a daughter.

This is not the most helpful response. This response reflects the husband's experience. It communicates to Mr. Biener that the nurse understands that he has a daughter, but this is not particularly helpful. Both parties now know the sex of Mr. Biener's new child, but the nurse's response, by ignoring Mr. Biener's thoughts and feelings about his new daughter, does not communicate understanding of the rest of Mr. Biener's message.

A response that reflects the patient's feelings is always more helpful than one that does not. It is up to the listener to decide whether reflection of the speaker's experience and/or thoughts in *addition* to reflection of the speaker's feelings will prove helpful.

A response that reflects both Mr. Biener's feelings and his experience would be the most helpful. It would include reference to his joy and to his new daughter.

Return to page 91 and pick out the most helpful response.

You picked B

You got your wish. You wanted a daughter because you already have two sons.

This is not the most helpful response. This response reflects Mr. Biener's experience. It communicates to him that the nurse understands his desire for a daughter and his recent fulfillment of that desire. However, this response is not sufficient in itself, because it ignores Mr. Biener's thoughts and feelings about his new daughter. It's often a difficult distinction to make, but Mr. Biener's statement that "We wanted a little girl more than anything" is really a statement of an experience. It's an expression of a past desire—something that Mr. and Mrs. Biener experienced in the past. (If this statement were in the present tense, it would be classified as a thought.)

A response that reflects the speaker's feelings is frequently helpful. It's up to the nurse to decide whether reflection of the speaker's experiences and/or thoughts *in addition* to reflection of the speaker's feelings will prove helpful.

A response that reflects Mr. Biener's feelings and his experience would be the most helpful. It would include reference to his joy and to his new daughter.

Return to page 91 and pick out the most helpful response.

You picked C

You feel wonderful. You got the daughter you wanted.

Congratulations! This response is the most helpful one. It reflects both Mr. Biener's feelings and his experience. It communicates to him that the nurse understands his happiness and the reason for it. This response is also short; therefore it immediately turns the focus to Mr. Biener, allowing him to further express his happiness if he wishes to do so.

Notice that Mr. Biener's original statement contained only one expression of affect: "I feel great." All three statements, "We had a daughter," "We already have two sons, Tom and Mike," and "We wanted a little girl more than anything," are all classified as experiences. The first two report observable events, and the last statement reports a previously experienced desire. If this desire were unfulfilled and stated in the present tense, it would be classified as a thought.

Turn to page 95.

Selective Responding: Exercise 2

Read the following statement and decide which of the responses is the most helpful.

> **Mrs. Johnson:** *It's all over. I know it. I'll never leave this hospital again. I'm scared.*
>
> **Nurse Responses:** A. *You're frightened.*
> B. *You're afraid you're going to die.*
> C. *You think you're never going to leave this hospital again.*

If you picked A, turn to page 96.
If you picked B, turn to page 97.
If you picked C, turn to page 98.

You picked A

You're frightened.

This is not the most helpful response. This response reflects only Mrs. Johnson's feelings. By ignoring all the other components of her statement, it might inadvertently pressure her into further expression of feeling. It communicates to her that you understand her fear, but it does not express an understanding of why she is afraid.

A response that reflects both her thoughts and her feelings would be more helpful. It would communicate interest in what the patient is thinking as well as in how she is feeling. This would allow Mrs. Johnson to elaborate on her original statement in either of these two areas, rather than pressure her to further disclose her feelings.

A more helpful response than the one you chose would be one that reflects the patient's thoughts about the possibility of her recovery as well as her feelings of fear.

Return to page 95 and pick out the most helpful response.

You picked B

> ***You're afraid you're going to die.***

Congratulations! This is the most helpful response. It reflects both Mrs. Johnson's thoughts and her feelings. It doesn't pressure her into a further expression of feelings but does communicate interest both in what she is thinking and in how she is feeling.

Notice that response A, "You're frightened," reflects the patient's feelings and ignores her thoughts, and response C, "You think you're never going to leave this hospital again," reflects the patient's thoughts but ignores her feelings.

Turn to page 99.

You picked C

You think you're never going to leave this hospital again.

This is not the most helpful response. It reflects Mrs. Johnson's thoughts but ignores her feelings. It might communicate to her that the nurse is interested in Mrs. Johnson's analysis of her physical condition but that the nurse is afraid of the intensity of the patient's feelings.

A response that reflects the patient's thoughts and her feelings would be more helpful. It would communicate interest both in what the patient is thinking and in how she is feeling. It would invite the patient to further express herself in either of these two areas.

A more helpful response than the one you chose would reflect this patient's feelings of fear as well as her pessimistic prediction about her recovery.

Return to page 95 and try again.

Selective Responding: Exercise 3

Read the following statement and decide which of the responses is the most helpful.

Mr. Gasser: *You know that it's costing me $120 a day just to lie in this bed. It makes me mad as hell! You people act like I'm made of money. You know I don't have insurance!*

Nurses Responses: A. *You feel angry that this illness is costing you so much money.*

B. *Since you don't have insurance, it's costing you $120 a day to be here.*

C. *You're mad because you don't have insurance.*

If you picked A, turn to page 100.
If you picked B, turn to page 101.
If you picked C, turn to page 102.

You picked A

> **You feel angry that this illness is costing you so much money.**

Congratulations! This is the most helpful response. It reflects Mr. Gasser's anger and his thoughts related to that anger. It communicates to him that the nurse understands his emotional state and the reason for it. It invites him to talk further about the high hospital costs or about his feelings related to those costs. The single phrase "This illness is costing you so much money" briefly paraphrases both of these statements by Mr. Gasser: "You know that it's costing me $120 a day just to lie in this bed" and "You know I don't have insurance!"

Notice that response B, "Since you don't have insurance, it's costing you $120 a day to be here," ignores the patient's anger and that response C. "You're mad because you don't have insurance," draws an uncertain parallel between Mr. Gasser's anger and his lack of insurance. This last response also ignores the patient's statement that "You people act like I'm made of money." This criticism, which is not directed at any particular person, is tangential to the major problem expressed.

By making a reflective response, the nurse does not have to defend the high cost of medical care and can simply listen to the patient's complaints.

Turn to page 103.

You picked B

Since you don't have insurance, it's costing you $120 a day to be here.

This is not the most helpful response. It reflects the statements "You know that it's costing me $120 a day just to lie in this bed" and "You know I don't have insurance!" However, it ignores Mr. Gasser's anger. This response might communicate to Mr. Gasser that, although the nurse understands how much he is being charged for his hospital stay, the nurse is afraid of his anger about it.

A response that reflects both the patient's feelings and his experiences would be more helpful. It's up to the nurse to paraphrase the speaker's feelings in an intensity similar to that with which they were presented and to paraphrase any other statements that seem central to the patient's feelings and essential to communicating understanding of the patient.

A response that reflects Mr. Gasser's feelings and experience would be the most helpful. It would include reference to his anger and to its cause.

Return to page 99 and pick out the most helpful response.

You picked C

You're mad because you don't have insurance.

This is not the most helpful response. It reflects the statements "It makes me mad as hell!" and "You know I don't have insurance!" but it links the two statements in a cause-and-effect relationship that was not mentioned by the patient. Mr. Gasser is not mad at the fact that he does not have insurance but at the expensive hospital costs he will have to pay because he doesn't have insurance. If he was mad because he didn't have insurance, his anger would be directed partially at himself because he was responsible for the decision not to purchase insurance. The fact that Mr. Gasser's statements begin with phrases such as "You know" and "You people" is a clue that his anger is directed at others.

A response that reflects both the patient's feelings and his experiences would be more helpful. It's up to the nurse to paraphrase both the speaker's feelings and any other statements that seem central to his feelings and essential to communicating understanding of the patient.

A response that reflects Mr. Gasser's feelings and experience would be most helpful. It would include reference to his anger and to its cause.

Return to page 99 and pick out the most helpful response.

Selective Responding: Exercise 4

Read the following statement by a patient and then write three reflective responses. The first should reflect only the content of the patient's message. It should reflect both the patient's experience and his thoughts but should ignore the patient's feelings. The second should reflect only the patient's feelings. It should ignore the content of the patient's message. The third should reflect both the content and the feelings expressed in the patient's message.

> **Stan:** *That was my sister Jo Ann who just left. I haven't seen her in years. She came all the way from Salt Lake City to visit me. I feel wonderful just seeing her again.*

Reflection of content:

Reflection of feelings:

Reflection of content and feelings:

Turn to the next page to check your answers.

There are a number of possible reflections for Stan's statement. Here are three sample responses that fulfill the criteria outlined. Your responses should parallel these.

Stan: *That was my sister Jo Ann who just left, I haven't seen her in years. She came all the way from Salt Lake City to visit me. I feel wonderful just seeing her again.*

Reflection of content:

Your sister, whom you haven't seen in years, came to visit you.

Reflection of feelings:

You feel happy.

Reflection of content and feelings:

You feel happy because your sister Jo Ann came all the way from Salt Lake City to visit you.

Proceed to the next page.

Selective Responding: Exercise 5

Read the following statement by a patient and then write three reflective responses as indicated.

> **George:**   *My leg—it hurts, it feels like it's on fire. I can't take the pain. I'm scared! Help me.*

Reflection of content:

Reflection of feelings:

Reflection of content and feelings:

Turn to the next page to check your answers.

Below are some sample reflective responses that selectively reflect the various components of George's message. Your responses should be similar to these.

> **George: *My leg—it hurts. It feels like it's on fire. I can't take the pain. I'm scared! Help me.***

Reflection of content:

> *You have a burning pain in your leg.*

Reflection of feelings:

> *You're frightened.*

Reflection of content and feelings:

> *Your leg is in so much pain that it's frightening.*

Proceed to the next page.

Selective Responding: Exercise 6

Read the following statement by a patient and then write three reflective responses as indicated.

Lynn: *I lost my baby. I can't stand it—I don't want to go on living! I feel empty inside.*

Reflection of content:

Reflection of feelings:

Reflection of content and feelings:

Turn to the next page to check your answers.

Here are some sample responses that selectively reflect various components of the patient's message. Your responses should be similar to these.

> **Lynn: I lost my baby. I can't stand it—I don't want to go on living! I feel empty inside.**

Reflection of content:

> *You lost your child.*

Reflection of feelings:

> *You feel empty—like you don't want to go on living.*

Reflection of content and feelings:

> *You feel like dying because your child is dead.*

Proceed to the next page.

THE PATIENT'S RESPONSE TO THE
NURSE'S REFLECTIONS

The reflective response is central to facilitative listening. It's a *selective response,* because the nurse does not paraphrase all the material presented by the patient. Instead, the nurse paraphrases what she or he considers to be of most vital importance in the message. The nurse can choose to respond to the feelings, to the content (experience and thoughts), or to both. Which of these the nurse reflects influences the direction of the next statement by the patient.

A response that reflects the patient's feelings is most likely to be followed by the patient with a further exploration of his or her feelings. By reflecting the patient's feelings, the nurse is actively demonstrating interest in them. This interest is reinforcing to the speaker and will encourage him or her to expand on those feelings. Here is an example of an interaction in which the nurse responded only to the patient's feelings.

Mr. Underhill: I'm so mad at that doctor! He didn't show up this morning to sign my discharge papers.

Nurse: You're angry at your doctor.

Mr. Underhill: Sure I'm angry! I'd like to see *him* stay in bed all day and wait for *me.*

This nurse selectively responded to Mr. Underhill's feelings of anger and in so doing signaled him that this aspect of his statement was accepted as significant. This reinforcement by the nurse will lead to further pursuit of this line of communication by Mr. Underhill. A response that reflects only the content of the patient's message and ignores the patient's feelings reinforces the reflected component and extinguishes the other component. This type of response increases the probability that the patient will ignore his or her feelings and expand on the content of the original message instead. For example, if the nurse responded to only the content of Mr. Underhill's statement, Mr. Underhill would probably talk further about his thoughts and experiences and ignore his own feelings of anger. Here is an example of one possible interaction.

Mr. Underhill: I'm so mad at that doctor! He didn't show up this morning to sign my discharge papers.

Nurse: You want to go home today, but Dr. Penn hasn't shown up yet to sign your discharge papers.

Mr. Underhill: He promised me yesterday he'd be in this morning. Today's my son's birthday, and I wanted to be home this morning to celebrate it with him.

Notice that this time the patient did not elaborate on his anger but chose to follow the nurse's cue and expand on the circumstances surrounding his anger. Occasionally a nurse will ignore the patient's expressed feelings but the patient will still choose to expand on those feelings. Such an occurrence indicates that the feelings expressed were both very present and very important to the speaker. Just having the nurse listen to any part of the message is encouragement enough for the patient to keep speaking.

Finally, a response that reflects both the content and the feelings expressed in the patient's message provides the patient with greater freedom of response. A good response by a nurse need not reflect the entire message of the patient; only the patient's feelings and the significant content related to those feelings need be related. A response that reflects both these components communicates to the patient that the nurse understands both how the patient feels and why she or he feels that way. It invites the patient to further explore either the thoughts or the feelings expressed. Consider the example of Mr. Underhill again.

Mr. Underhill: I'm so mad at that doctor! He didn't show up this morning to sign my discharge papers.

Nurse: You're mad at Dr. Penn because he hasn't shown up yet to sign your discharge papers.

Mr. Underhill: Mad? I'm steaming! Today's my son's birthday, and I wanted to spend the day with him.

Notice how Mr. Underhill acknowledged his feelings of anger and further explained his reasons for them. Since the nurse responded to—and thus reinforced—both his thoughts and his feelings, Mr. Underhill had the option of expanding on either or both of these components.

Responses that reflect both the thoughts and the feelings of a speaker are the most helpful. They provide the patient with the greatest freedom of response and give the patient greater control over the tempo of his or her disclosure. Responses that reflect only the content of the patient's statement and ignore the patient's expressed feelings are least helpful. They ignore the greatest disclosure in the message—the part that is central to the patient. Continuous reflection only of content will communicate that the expression of feeling is unacceptable. This discourages further expression of feelings by the patient. Responses that reflect only the patient's feelings can be helpful, but they carry with them the expectation or demand that the patient further explore these feelings. This can be threatening to the patient, because his or her feelings are the most revealing and personal disclosure that can be made. The patient may not wish to elaborate on them any further. Another danger in reflecting only feelings is that the patient must assure that the nurse heard the content of the message, even though it wasn't reflected. This assumption may or may not be accurate.

Patient's Responding: Exercise 1

In the following dialogue between a nurse and a patient, how is the patient likely to respond?

> **Mrs. Nava:** *I don't want my husband to see me like this. I'm afraid of losing him. With only one breast, I'm only half a woman.*
>
> **Nurse:** *You don't want to see your husband. You're afraid he'll reject you.*
>
> **Mrs. Nava:** A. *What time are visiting hours?*
>
> B. *A woman with one breast is not a woman.*
>
> C. *I'm afraid he won't say anything. He'll just stare at me when I need him to say that everything's all right. His silence will hurt too much.*

If you picked A, turn to page 113.
If you picked B, turn to page 114.
If you picked C, turn to page 115.

You picked A

What time are visiting hours?

This is not the most likely response. It's possible that Mrs. Nava would ask when visiting hours are if she is trying to decide what she's going to do when her husband arrives. However, if she's focusing on the nurse's response, this is not the most likely response. Mrs. Nava's original message contained an honest expression of both her thoughts and her feelings. The nurse in this case did a beautiful job of reflecting the patient's feelings and related thoughts. Mrs. Nava will most likely respond to the understanding communicated by the nurse and continue to express her feelings and thoughts.

Return to page 112 and pick the correct response.

You picked B

A woman with one breast is not a woman.

This is not the most likely response. Although it's possible that Mrs. Nava would repeat her thoughts concerning women who have had breast surgery if she's focusing on her internal reaction, it is not the most likely response if she is focusing on the nurse's response. The nurse ignored a similar statement made earlier by Mrs. Nava ("With only one breast, I'm only half a woman"). The patient's original message contained an honest expression of both her thoughts and her feelings. The nurse in this case did a beautiful job of reflecting Mrs. Nava's feelings and related thoughts. Mrs. Nava will most likely respond to the understanding communicated by the nurse and continue to express her feelings and her thoughts.

Return to page 112 and pick the correct response.

You picked C

> *I'm afraid he won't say anything. He'll just stare at me when I need him to say that everything's all right. His silence will hurt too much.*

This is the most likely response. The other two responses are possible; however, if Mrs. Nava is focusing on the nurse's responses, response C is the most likely. Mrs. Nava's original message contained an honest expression of her thoughts ("I don't want my husband to see me like this. With only one breast, I'm only half a woman") and her feelings ("I'm afraid of losing him"). The nurse reflected Mrs. Nava's feelings and related thoughts and ignored the statement "With only one breast, I'm only half a woman." Mrs. Nava is likely to respond to the understanding communicated by the nurse and respond by expanding on her feelings and thoughts.

Turn to page 116.

Patient's Responding: Exercise 2

In the following dialogue between a nurse and a patient, how is the patient likely to respond?

> *Mr. Howard:*   *I'm nervous just lying here. I worry about taking care of my family. I have to earn money so they can live, and I can't keep missing work.*
>
> *Nurse: You're worried about your family and how they're going to manage without your income.*
>
> *Mr. Howard:*   A. *I don't know what's going to happen. I might lose my job, and then what would I do?*
>
>   B. *I wonder how they're managing. I worry that they don't have enough money to live on but that they don't tell me.*
>
>   C. *I'm a carpenter, you know. Been with the same company for 20 years. My boss told me not to worry, but I can't help it.*

If you picked A, turn to page 117.
If you picked B, turn to page 118.
If you picked C, turn to page 119.

You picked A

> *I don't know what's going to happen. I might lose my job, and then what would I do?*

This is not the most likely response. In Mr. Howard's original statement, he expressed his thoughts and feelings concerning the lack of income caused by his hospitalization and the effect that it might be having on his family. The nurse reflected his feelings of concern about his family but ignored his statement about his job. Mr. Howard will probably not expand on the thoughts ignored by the nurse. Instead, he will probably expand on his feelings about his family and their financial crisis.

Return to page 116 and select the most helpful response.

You picked B

> *I wonder how they're managing. I worry that they don't have enough money to live on but that they don't tell me.*

This is the most likely response. Mr. Howard's original statement contains an honest expression of both his thoughts ("I have to earn money so they can live, and I can't keep missing work") and his feelings ("I'm nervous just lying here. I worry about taking care of my family"). The nurse responded to Mr. Howard's thoughts and feelings and related to his concern for his family's well-being. She ignored his statement about his job. Mr. Howard will probably respond to the nurse's interest in his family by expanding on these thoughts and feelings.

Turn to page 120.

You picked C

I'm a carpenter, you know. Been with the same company for 20 years. My boss told me not to worry, but I can't help it.

This is not the most likely response. In Mr. Howard's original statement, he expressed his thoughts and feelings concerning the lack of income caused by his hospitalization and the effect that it has on his family. The nurse ignored his statement related to work ("I can't keep missing work"). Response C is an extension of that statement about his work. It is unlikely that Mr. Howard would make such a statement after the nurse ignored his original reference to his work. He would be more likely to expand on his feelings related to his family and their financial crisis.

Return to page 116 and select the most likely response.

Patient's Responding: Exercise 3

In the following dialogue between a nurse and a patient, how is the patient likely to respond?

> **Mrs. Steinberg:** *My son's really sick. They want me to leave him here until the end of the week for tests. I don't know if I can live without him. I'm scared.*
>
> **Nurse:** *They want you to leave your son here for more tests.*
>
> **Mrs. Steinberg:** A. *I don't know if I can leave him. He's never been away from home before, and I'm so used to having him around.*
>
> B. *Yeah. They want to give him a whole battery of tests. I don't even remember what they called them—something to do with his blood.*
>
> C. *I don't know what's going to happen. I'm in a state of shock from this whole thing. I'm just scared stiff.*

If you picked A, turn to page 121.
If you picked B, turn to page 122.
If you picked C, turn to page 123.

You picked A

I don't know if I can leave him. He's never been away from home before, and I'm so used to having him around.

This is not the most likely response. Mrs. Steinberg's original statement contained experiential, cognitive, and affective components. The nurse's response ignored Mrs. Steinberg's thoughts and feelings and reflected only the observable event reported by the patient. The most likely response by the patient is a continued expression of the event reflected by the nurse. In response A, Mrs. Steinberg again reports an experience ("He's never been away from home before") and expands on her thoughts ("I don't know if I can leave him. . . . I'm so used to having him around"). This response is unlikely, since Mrs. Steinberg's original response contained a similar statement ("I don't know if I can live without him"), which was ignored by the nurse. She will probably be influenced by the nurse's response to discontinue this line of communication.

Although Mrs. Steinberg is willing to share her doubts and her feelings of fear with the nurse, she will most likely stop doing so, because the nurse ignored her initial expressions in these areas. Mrs. Steinberg is more likely to expand on the idea of leaving her son in the hospital for more tests.

Return to page 120 and pick out the correct response.

You picked B

> *Yeah. They want to give him a whole battery of tests. I don't even remember what they called them—something to do with his blood.*

This is the most likely response. Mrs. Steinberg's original statement contained an experiential component ("My son's really sick. They want me to leave him here until the end of the week for tests"), a cognitive component ("I don't know if I can live without him"), and an affective component ("I'm scared"). The nurse's response ("They want you to leave your son here for more tests") ignored both the cognitive and the affective components of the message. Mrs. Steinberg's most likely response is to follow the nurse's lead, ignoring her doubts and feelings of fear and continuing to expand the experiential component of the message. In response B she does just that.

Turn to page 124.

You picked C

I don't know what's going to happen. I'm in a state of shock from this whole thing. I'm just scared stiff.

This is not the most likely response. Mrs. Steinberg's original statement contained an experiential, a cognitive, and an affective component. The nurse's response ignored the patient's thoughts and feelings and paraphrased only the experiential component of her message. The most likely patient response is a continued expression of the experiences reflected by the nurse. In response C, the patient does not express observable events; she expresses her feelings.

Although Mrs. Steinberg is willing to share her feelings of fear with the nurse, she will most likely stop doing so, because the nurse ignored her initial attempt at affective expression. Mrs. Steinberg will most likely expand on the idea of leaving her son in the hospital for more tests.

Return to page 120 and pick out the correct response.

CONSEQUENCES OF REFLECTIVE LISTENING

Now that you've learned the basic components of the reflective response, what are some obvious consequences you should expect if you use such a response?

First, if you employ this listening skill, the first thing you should notice is that the *patient talks more.* A reflective listener is a constant encouragement to any speaker. Showing interest in what is said causes the patient to express himself or herself more thoroughly.

Second, since the reflective listener neither passes judgment on the speaker nor offers solutions, *the patient is not threatened by the reflective listener.* This reduction of external threat causes the patient to explore and express himself or herself more deeply. You'll notice that the patient is opening up more.

Third, you will realize that *you do not always hear as accurately as you thought you did.* Many times after you give a reflective response, the patient will say "No, that's not what I mean. What I wanted to say was . . ." You'll realize that your listening is biased by your perceptions and that you don't always hear what is said.

Fourth, *the patient will realize that his or her communication is not always as clear as she or he might like it to be.*

Fifth, *you will understand people better* than you ever have in the past, because you will be checking out your perceptions with them. This deeper understanding will make you realize how much you "missed" before of what was being said to you.

Sixth, *you will come to understand that you play as great a role in interactions when you are an active listener as you do when you are a speaker.* Listening is a positive reinforcer, and with it you can influence the speaker.

Last, *you will feel more satisfied in your interactions with others,* because, instead of two people throwing thoughts at each other, one person is giving and the other is receiving. A conversational flow is established, rather than the clash of colliding statements.

The reflective response is central to active listening. However, it is not without its drawbacks, especially when overused or abused to the point of "parroting" responses. For example, a woman who has just learned the reflective response might have the following conversation with her husband.

Husband: I'm certainly in the mood for a steak dinner tonight.

Wife: You certainly would like to have a steak tonight.

Husband (at the restaurant): This is a great steak.

Wife: You're really enjoying that steak.

Husband: Would you pass the salt, please?

Wife: You would like me to pass you the salt.

Husband: What on earth is wrong with you!

Understandably, the husband is upset, because continuous
reflective responses would be difficult for anyone to deal with,
especially when shallow content matter is being reflected.

Good reflective responses are more difficult to give than
it might at first appear. Nurses who are just learning how to
respond reflectively stand out among more experienced listeners, because they tend to repeat the patient's message almost
word for word. This verbatim repetition causes the patient to
wonder what's going on, and she or he will often confront the
nurse with questions such as "Don't you hear very well?" and
"Why do you keep telling me what I just told you?" Such responses on the part of the patient do not violate the
usefulness of the technique; they only demonstrate that the
listener is inexperienced. Reflection sounds like a mere
technique—and indeed it can be if it has not been incorporated by the beginner as a part of his or her verbal repertoire.
Experience will facilitate incorporation, and knowledge and
practice of other response patterns will prevent overuse and
misuse of the reflective response.

6
Clarification

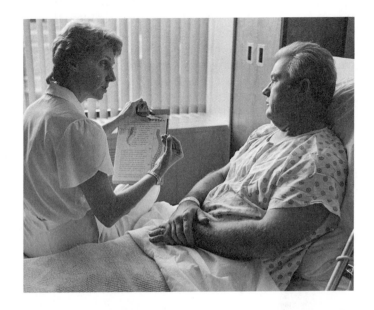

BASIC CLARIFICATION RESPONSES

Now that you've mastered the reflective response, you can refine your communication skills by learning to use the clarification response. The clarifying listener assumes the internal frame of reference of the speaker and attempts to understand what the patient is thinking and feeling by placing himself or herself in the patient's shoes. The clarifying listener communicates understanding by *elaborating* on the thoughts and feelings of the speaker. Whereas the reflective listener repeats the content of the original statement, only responding to what was actually said by the patient, the clarifying listener amplifies the patient's statement, responding to what is not said as well as to what is said. By clarifying what the patient has said, the clarifying listener expands both the feeling and the content expressed. In this way the clarifying listener helps the patient to better understand himself or herself.

Clarifications are phrased in terms of the patient and might begin with phrases such as "You feel as though" or "At times it seems to you that." During clarification the focus remains on the patient, with the listener attempting to express feelings at a level deeper and in more detail than the patient is able to express. The aim is to help the patient to acknowledge and express these feelings.

The clarifying listener does not interpret the patient's messages. She or he does not add any new information to the comments of the patient; rather, the listener's comments are based on the previous expressions of the patient. The clarifying listener expands the comments of the patient rather than interprets them. Interpreting the speaker's message would involve adding new content and feelings to the expressions of the patient—content and feeling that are not based on the previous expressions of the patient but that are projections concerning the patient. Interpretations are risky, because they attribute motive and feelings to the patient that are not necessarily his or her own. Incorrect interpretations communicate a lack of understanding, and correct ones are often frightening to the patient, because they involve content and feelings that are understood by the listener but that the patient has not yet chosen to share. Generally, patients prefer to have their comments accepted as they are given rather than examined for hidden meaning.

While working with patients, try to come to understand their behavior without interpretations. Clarify their comments so that they can come to better understand themselves, but avoid categorizing patients and offering your projections about the reasons for their behavior. Try to be helpful. Listen to what the patient says without asking yourself why he or she said it. Try to master the clarification response; it should prove immensely helpful.

Examine the following clarification by a nurse.

Mr. Birchall: It's my wife, she's dying. I'm afraid to go in there and see her. I can't act cheerful, and it won't do her any good to see me upset.

Nurse Clarification: You feel concerned about your wife, but you think her seeing your sadness will only aggravate her condition. You're afraid of what might happen to her because of your upset.

Notice that the nurse in her response focused on the speaker and his feelings, phrasing the response in terms of him. The nurse used statements such as "you feel" to underline this focus. The only feeling the speaker expressed was his fear of visiting his wife. The nurse, by integrating his or her knowledge of the speaker and of how he or she would feel in a similar situation, surmised that the speaker felt nervous and uncomfortable. However, the nurse might be wrong in this projection of why the speaker doesn't want to see his wife. The nurse's assumption will be verified or discounted when the speaker responds to the nurse's clarification.

Look at this clarification of an earlier patient statement.

Florence Greene: I've been ringing this call bell for 20 minutes and no one has bothered to answer. What are you running here, a hospital or a social club for nurses?

Mr. Bradley: You're angry because the staff hasn't responded to your call as quickly as you think they should.

In this statement the patient expresses her experience and her thoughts related to that experience. The patient's sarcasm implies that she's angry, but she does not state these feelings overtly. The nurse immediately focuses on these unexpressed feelings of anger, communicating to the patient "I hear you, and it's OK for you to feel the way you do." By using his understanding of the patient's thoughts and implied feelings, the nurse assumes that the reason for the patient's anger is that the staff didn't respond to her summons as quickly as the patient thought they should. This may or may not be a correct assumption.

Clarifying: Exercise 1

A 17-year-old patient, Melissa, made the following statement to the nurse. Which of the responses is an example of clarification?

> **Melissa:**   *I'm having a terrible time with my doctor. She hates me. Is there anything you can do?*
>
> **Ms. Rostow:**   A. *You think your doctor hates you, and you want to know if there's anything I can do to remedy the situation.*
>
> B. *Before I started working with doctors, I was uncomfortable around them, too. I thought they were too busy to talk to me.*
>
> C. *You're concerned about your relationship with your doctor. You think she doesn't like you, and it's getting you down.*

If you picked A, turn to page 132.
If you picked B, turn to page 133.
If you picked C, turn to page 134.

You picked A

You think your doctor hates you, and you want to know if there's anything I can do to remedy the situation.

Close, but not quite. You were to pick an example of clarification, which develops the thoughts and feelings of the patient. Response A does not amplify the thoughts and feelings of the patient; it merely restates the original problem in different words.

This response is a reflective one. Both reflection and clarification focus on the patient and try to demonstrate an understanding of the original statement, but there is a difference. The reflective listener does not amplify the original statement; the clarifying listener adds his or her perceptions and insights to try to help the patient better understand himself or herself. This expanded content usually focuses on what the listener perceives the patient to be feeling. The listener shares these perceptions with the patient, and in his or her next response the speaker can either verify or deny these perceptions.

A clarifying response would expand the thoughts and/or feelings already expressed by Melissa. The clarifying listener would try to show Melissa that she really understands how Melissa is feeling.

Return to page 131 and try again to pick out the correct response.

You picked B

Before I started working with doctors, I was uncomfortable around them, too. I thought they were too busy to talk to me.

This is not the correct response. Let's see what happened. You were to pick an example of clarification, but the response you chose is an example of identification. The nurse involved is relating an experience similar to this patient's, hoping to show that she understands how Melissa feels. The focus is on the nurse and her experience.

A clarifying response focuses on the speaker and the speaker's experience. If this nurse were using clarification, he would attempt to show Melissa that he understands how she feels by sharing with her his perception of how she is feeling. The clarifying listener shares not his or her own experiences of feelings but his or her thoughts about how the speaker is feeling. Clarifying listeners try to put themselves in the speaker's shoes and then express how it feels to be in those shoes. Clarifying responses often fit the format of "you feel..., because..." A clarifying response would expand the thoughts and feelings already expressed by Melissa. The clarifying nurse would try to show Melissa that he really understands how she is feeling.

Return to page 131 and pick out the correct response.

You picked C

You're concerned about your relationship with your doctor. You think she doesn't like you, and it's getting you down.

Absolutely correct. This is an example of a clarifying response. There are many possible clarifying responses to the original statement. The nurse in this response tries to help the patient understand herself and the feelings she is experiencing. The clarifying listener elaborates on the original patient statement. The nurse focused on Melissa's concern and bad feelings about her relationship with her doctor. The patient did not directly express these feelings; they were sensed by the nurse. A clarifying response shifts the focus of the conversation from external events to feelings. The nurse is helping the patient not only to better understand herself but also to express her feelings more openly.

Turn to page 135.

Clarifying: Exercise 2

A 70-year-old male patient, Andrew Henderson, makes the following statement to the staff nurse as she enters the room. Which of the responses is an example of clarification?

> **Andrew Henderson:** *I saw you in there with all the other nurses. Were you talking about me? I know I'm a problem.*

> **Mrs. Farley:** A. *What other nurses was I talking with when you saw me?*
>
> B. *You're worried that I was talking about you to some of the other nurses. You think your behavior would give us reason to talk about you, and you wonder what was said.*
>
> C. *Often when I see two of my friends talking, I wonder whether they're talking about me. When I know I've done something to hurt either of them, I feel guilty and my suspicions are even stronger.*

If you picked A, turn to page 136.
If you picked B, turn to page 137.
If you picked C, turn to page 138.

You picked A

What other nurses was I talking with when you saw me?

You were to pick an example of clarification. Instead, you picked a question. A question asks the patient to elaborate on an experience, on thoughts, or on feelings. The response you selected asked the patient to expand on his description of the experience. Clarification does involve expanding on the patient's experience, thoughts, and feelings, but the nurse is the one who does the expanding. Usually the nurse elaborates on the patient's feelings. By sensing how the patient feels, focusing on these feelings, and sharing this focus with the patient, the nurse gives Mr. Henderson more insight into his own behavior and feelings.

A clarifying response would focus on Mr. Henderson's feelings of worry and wonder. He did not overtly express either of these feelings, yet both were implied. The clarifying nurse would try to help the patient better understand the reason for his feelings in this situation.

Return to page 135 and try to pick out the example of clarification.

You picked B

You're worried that I was talking about you to some of the other nurses. You think your behavior would give us reason to talk about you, and you wonder what was said.

Good for you. Notice that the nurse here focused on the patient's feelings—worry and wonder. The clarifying nurse tries to help the patient to better understand his feelings in this situation, although neither his worry nor his wonder was overtly expressed. This response attempted to give him insight into his feelings and their cause as well as demonstrated the intensity of the nurse's listening and understanding.

Turn to page 139.

You picked C

> *Often when I see two of my friends talking, I wonder*
> *whether they're talking about me. When I know I've done*
> *something to hurt either of them, I feel guilty and my*
> *suspicions are even stronger.*

You were to pick an example of clarification. This is not it. This is an example of identification. This response is phrased in terms of the nurse. She is talking in the first person about herself and uses phrases such as "I feel," "I wonder," and "I think." The nurse is relating not only Mr. Henderson's thoughts and feelings about his experience but also her own personal experience.

A clarifying response is phrased in terms of the patient and expands what the patient has already said. The clarifying listener talks in the second person, using such phrases as "you feel," "you wonder," and "you think." The nurse would focus on the implied feelings of the patient—curiosity and guilt. She would tell the patient why he was experiencing these feelings.

Return to page 135 and try again to pick out the example of clarification.

Clarifying: Exercise 3

Given the following patient statement, which of the following responses by the nurse is an example of clarification?

Joel Thompson: *Every morning when the nurse comes in to give me a shot, he shakes me to wake me up. I hate it. I wish he'd just leave me alone and give me the shot when I get up by myself.*

Ms. Xavier: A. *You really feel angry at the nurse. You wish he was less persistent in giving you medication prescribed for you.*
   B. *You hate having the nurse shake you when he wakes you up in the morning.*
   C. *I feel terrible for you. The morning nurse should know better than to do that.*

If you picked A, turn to page 140.
If you picked B, turn to page 141.
If you picked C, turn to page 142.

You picked A

You really feel angry at the nurse. You wish he was less persistent in giving you the medication prescribed for you.

Great! You picked the correct response. This response is an example of clarification because the nurse expanded the original statement of the patient. She perceived that the patient was angry at the nurse for his behavior and shared this perception with the patient, although Joel did not directly express this anger in his original statement. It is to be hoped that this clarification of his feelings will enable Joel to express his anger and deal with it. The nurse also expanded the patient's thoughts related to his feelings.

Turn to page 143.

You picked B

You hate having the nurse shake you when he wakes you up in the morning.

This is not the correct response. You were to pick an example of clarification, and this response illustrates reflection. It focuses on the patient and his feelings, but it only restates what the patient has already said. The patient's statement is expressed in slightly different words and the sequence is changed, but the message is essentially the same.

A clarifying response has a message that is different from that of the original statement. New material is added. A clarifying listener shares with the patient what she or he thinks the patient is feeling. The response you chose merely restates what the patient said. It focuses on the patient's expressed dislike for the nurse's behavior. The correct response would focus on the patient's anger and his reaction to the morning medication.

Return to page 139 and try to pick out the example of clarification.

You picked C

> ***I feel terrible for you. The morning nurse should know better than to do that.***

This is not the correct response. It contains a personal expression of affect by the nurse. She is telling the patient how she feels about another nurse's behavior and in doing so is passing judgment on that behavior. The nurse's response focuses on what she thinks and feels, rather than on what the patient thinks and feels.

The correct response would amplify the patient's thoughts and feelings. It would focus on the patient's anger and on his thoughts related to that anger.

Return to page 139 and try again.

RECOGNIZING IMPLIED THOUGHTS
AND FEELINGS

Clarification has been defined as a response that expands on what is not said as well as what is said. The clarifying listener amplifies and elaborates the comments of the patient. She or he adds deeper feeling and meaning to the expressions of the patient by responding not only to the expressed thoughts and feelings of the patient but also to the underlying ones.

All messages are composed of experiential, cognitive, and affective components. Any combination of these components can exist, yielding seven types of messages: messages containing (1) only an experiential component, (2) only a cognitive component, (3) only an affective component, (4) both an experiential and a cognitive component, (5) both an experiential and an affective component, (6) both a cognitive and an affective component, and (7) all three components. A clarifying listener can choose to elaborate on any combination of these components. Usually, the experiential and cognitive components are considered together as the content of the message. The nurse can choose to respond to the content, to the feelings, or to the content and the feelings.

The major focus of clarification is usually on the patient's feelings, because an understanding of the patient's feelings is crucial to understanding the patient. Most problems do concern feelings that, for some reason, are causing the patient difficulty. In order to help the patient understand and deal more constructively with troublesome feelings, the nurse must first help the patient express these feelings. By clarifying the patient's feelings, the nurse is helping the patient express them more openly. By focusing on the feelings and amplifying them, the nurse is showing the patient that she or he would like the patient to talk about them. The nurse who clarifies a patient's feelings is saying, "It's all right to talk about feelings here. I'd like you to share your feelings with me in as much detail as possible. I'll help you to do that by amplifying the feelings you express or imply."

The clarifying listener responds to feelings that are unstated as well as to those that are expressed. She or he listens and watches for clues that will help in understanding how the patient feels about the problem at hand. Clues as to how the patient feels can be either verbal or nonverbal. These clues are like pieces of a puzzle and, when put together, can reveal much about the patient. The clarifying listener makes assumptions about the meaning of these clues and shares those assumptions with the patient. Both what the patient says and how it is said provide verbal clues to his or her underlying feelings. Word choice, speech rate, intonation, and tonal quality all provide verbal clues to the feelings underlying the message. Verbal clues such as stammering, shouting, a quivering voice, and long pauses can be indications that a sensitive topic is being presented. The patient's physical behavior also provides clues to underlying feelings. The perceptive nurse will watch the speaker for any physical indications of nervousness or tension and will focus more attention on the areas of the conversation during which these occurred. Body posture, gestures, and the nature of the patient's movements all can provide the nurse with information about the patient. The nurse should be especially alert to changes in verbal and nonverbal behavior, because these changes provide clues to the areas of the interaction that the patient finds especially sensitive. If a patient's voice starts to quiver only when she talks about her mother, she probably has deeper feelings about this relationship than she has about other topics in the conversation.

The clarification response lets the patient know that you have heard these clues. It further tells him or her that you recognize the unexpressed thoughts and feelings that underlie the communication. It says "Here's what I think your unexpressed thoughts and feelings are. Am I right? If so, why don't you talk about them? If I'm wrong, please correct me."

Even though all messages do not contain overt expressions of feelings, all messages do contain unstated feelings. For now, the absence of feelings also will be defined as a feeling state—namely, that state in which the person has no feelings. The fact that a patient does not have any feelings about a situation is just as important as if he or she had very strong feelings about the situation.

There are many reasons why a patient would choose not to express any feelings when speaking to the nurse. Perhaps the most common of these is that the patient has never learned how to talk about feelings. In fact, many people have learned how not to talk about feelings. How often have you seen a patient try to share personal feelings, only to have the listener become uncomfortable? The listener can communicate this discomfort by gestures such as looking down at the floor, rather than at the speaker; by rapidly changing the focus of the conversation; or by making comments such as "You don't mean that." These all signal to the patient that the topic of conversation is inappropriate or unacceptable. These indications of discomfort are frequent when personal feelings are being conveyed. Thus, one of the major challenges to the nurse is to communicate to the patient that it is appropriate to share feelings and that it is desirable as well. The patient must learn that in this relationship there is a new set of rules and that expressions of a personal, revealing nature are welcome.

Another reason that feelings are often omitted is the patient's fear of the consequences of expressing them. Often patients are ashamed of their feelings and afraid that, if their feelings are expressed, the nurse will reject or look down on them. Patients ask themselves "How can you like me if I behave this way? I don't even like myself when I behave this way." Thus, the feelings the patient is ashamed of are compounded by feelings of shame or guilt at having such feelings. Removing the shame and guilt is the first step in helping the speaker accept his or her feelings as legitimate and acceptable.

The nurse is faced with a real challenge in this area. She or he must communicate to the patient an unfaltering respect so that the patient will feel free to express his or her feelings openly. This communication of respect says to the patient "I understand these feelings you are sharing with me, and I still respect you." This will help the patient to share more of himself or herself, because the nurse will have provided a nonthreatening environment for doing so. It will also help patients to accept themselves, because they will experience the nurse as accepting them with full knowledge of their feelings.

It is therefore important for the nurse to acknowledge and accept both the expressed and the unexpressed feelings of the patient. In order to respond to them, of course, she or he must first be aware of them. Consider the following patient statement:

Robert: I feel great! I get to go home tomorrow. With hard work, my leg should be as good as new in about six months. I'll even be able to play football again next season. My coach is really relieved.

Robert is openly stating that he feels terrific. However, other feelings are being implied. He feels *relief* because his leg will heal completely and *joy* because he'll get to play football again.

Recognizing Feelings: Exercise 1

Read the following patient statements and write down what you consider to be the expressed and implied feelings in each.

> *Quentin: I feel very worried about all these tests I'm supposed to have. I've never had any tests before. Do they hurt?*

Expressed feelings:

Implied feelings:

> *Isaac: I'm really excited about the way things are going here. It's amazing. I haven't felt dizzy for a week. Maybe someday soon I'll feel like my old self again.*

Expressed feelings:

Implied feelings:

Below are some possible verbalizations of the expressed and implied feelings contained in each patient statement. Synonyms for the feelings listed are also acceptable.

> ***Quentin:*** *I feel very worried about all these tests I'm supposed to have. I've never had any tests before. Do they hurt?*

Expressed feelings:

Worry

Implied feelings:

Fear

> ***Isaac:*** *I'm really excited about the way things are going here. It's amazing. I haven't felt dizzy for a week. Maybe someday soon I'll feel like my old self again.*

Expressed feelings:

Excitement

Implied feelings:

Hope, relief

Recognizing Feelings: Exercise 2

Read the following patient statement and write down what you consider to be the expressed and implied feelings.

> ***Anita Adams:*** *I feel very distant from my family, I don't know what's wrong with me. All of a sudden I can't communicate with anyone. We were all so close before, and now when I'm talking to them, I feel like I'm talking to strangers.*

Expressed feelings:

Implied feelings:

Below are some possible verbalizations of the expressed and implied feelings contained in the patient statement. Synonyms for the feeling listed are also acceptable.

> ***Anita Adams:*** *I feel very distant from my family. I don't know what's wrong with me. All of a sudden I can't communicate with anyone. We were all so close before, and now when I'm talking to them, I feel like I'm talking to strangers.*

Expressed feelings:

Distance

Implied feelings:

Loneliness, concern, confusion

This patient expresses that she feels distant from her family both in her opening statement, "I feel very distant," and in her closing statement, "I feel like I'm talking to strangers." Throughout the communication is the unexpressed feeling of loneliness. Anita also feels confused—"I don't know what's wrong with me"—and concerned—"All of a sudden I can't communicate with anyone."

Recognizing Feelings: Exercise 3

Read the following patient statement and write down what you consider to be the expressed and implied feelings.

> **Diane York:** *I'm going to die. I just know it. I'm going to die! My whole life is over, and it hasn't even begun. It hasn't even begun!*

Expressed feelings:

Implied feelings:

Below are possible verbalizations of the expressed and implied feelings contained in the patient statement. Synonyms for the feelings listed are also acceptable.

> **Diane York: *I'm going to die. I just know it. I'm going to die! My whole life is over, and it hasn't even begun. It hasn't even begun!***

Expressed feelings:

(None)

Implied feelings:

Disappointment, anger

Diane did not express any feelings openly. Because of the highly personal nature of her disclosure, this is not unusual. She will probably wait to see how the nurse responds to her first statement before she decides whether to openly express her feelings. If the nurse responds with a statement that communicates avoidance or discomfort, Diane will probably not disclose her feelings. By acknowledging the feelings that are implied, the nurse can help Diane to express her feelings. Diane's repetition of the statement "It hasn't even begun" is a way of emphasizing that she feels disappointed and cheated because she's going to die. Diane undoubtedly has other feelings regarding her impending death, but there is no way to know what those feelings are until she discloses them.

Clarifying Feelings: Exercise 1

Read the following patient statements and identify the expressed and implied feelings. Then write a clarification response that attends to the patient's feelings.

> **Arnie:** I came to the hospital to feel better, but nothing you do here seems to do any good. I still feel terrible, and I still don't know what's wrong with me. I wish I could just feel good for a change.

Nurse's clarification of patient's feelings:

> **Oliver Klein:** I don't want to go home—not in this wheelchair anyhow. I can't manage without my legs.

Nurse's clarification of patient's feelings:

Below find possible clarification responses of the patient statements presented.

> **Arnie:**   **I came to the hospital to feel better but nothing you do here seems to do any good. I still feel terrible, and I still don't know what's wrong with me. I wish I could just feel good for a change.**

Nurse's clarification of patient's feelings:

> *You feel disappointed because nothing we do here seems to help you feel better.*

Correct responses should focus on the implied disappointment of the patient and the circumstances related to that disappointment.

> **Oliver Klein:**   **I don't want to go home—not in this wheelchair anyhow. I can't manage without my legs.**

Nurse's clarification of patient's feelings:

> *You're afraid to go home. You think you can't manage.*

Correct responses should focus on the patient's implied feeling of fear, shifting the reason for his desire not to go home from his statement "I don't want to" to his implied feeling "I'm afraid to." Notice also how this response changes the patient's statement "I can't manage" to "You think you can't manage."

Obviously, in addition to leaving out some of their feelings, patients many times do not tell the nurse all their thoughts. For whatever reason, patients usually keep some information from the nurse. Perhaps they think these thoughts are unimportant or too personal, or they may be embarrassed by some of their conclusions. Many times patients will allude to these unexpressed thoughts, giving the nurse a clue to what they are, because in some way the patients do want to share these thoughts. The nurse should be aware of clues, both verbal and nonverbal, that might help him or her to better understand the underlying thoughts of the patient. It is these unexpressed thoughts that can often reveal what is really going on with the patient.

In trying to listen for underlying thoughts, be understanding of the patient and try to put yourself in his or her place. Ask yourself what the patient must be thinking to feel the way he or she does. What assumptions does the patient hold that help facilitate this problem? Keep in mind that, even if the patient hasn't expressed any thoughts at all, underlying thoughts are still present. For example, note the implied thoughts in the following patient statement.

Florence Green: I've been ringing this call bell for 20 minutes and no one has bothered to answer. What are you running here, a hospital or a social club for nurses?

Notice that this patient expressed her thoughts sarcastically: "What are you running her, a hospital or a social club for nurses?" Her implied thoughts are "The staff members are not responding to my calls as quickly as they should" and "The staff is incompetent or negligent."

Recognizing Thoughts: Exercise 1

Read the following statements and write down what you consider to be the expressed and implied thoughts in each.

> **Peter Yost:**   *I don't feel any better now than I did before I started coming for treatments. In fact, I feel worse. It doesn't seem worth the effort.*

Expressed thoughts:

Implied thoughts:

> **Thomas Vale:**   *My hip is killing me. The medication you gave me at 3 o'clock isn't working anymore. I can't stand it.*

Expressed thoughts:

Implied thoughts:

Below are some possible statements of the expressed and implied thoughts in each of the patient statements.

> **Peter Yost:** *I don't feel any better now that I did before I started coming for treatments. In fact, I feel worse. It doesn't seem worth the effort.*

Expressed thoughts:

> *It doesn't seem worth the effort.*

Implied thoughts:

> *I should quit coming.*

> **Thomas Vale:** *My hip is killing me. The medication you gave me at 3 o'clock isn't working anymore. I can't stand it.*

Expressed thoughts:

> *I can't stand it.*

Implied thoughts:

> *I'd like to have more pain medication now.*

Recognizing Thoughts: Exercise 2

Read the following statement and write down what you consider to be the expressed and implied thoughts.

> *Richard Wilson: Listen, nurse, I want the truth from you. I ask everyone who comes in here what's wrong with me, and they all beat around the bush. One nurse says "What do you think is wrong?" and another tells me "Just be patient. Wait until the doctor arrives." Well, I'm tired of being patient. What's wrong with me?*

Expressed thoughts:

Implied thoughts:

Below are some possible statements of the expressed and implied thoughts contained in the patient's statement.

> ***Richard Wilson:*** *Listen, nurse, I want the truth from you. I ask everyone who comes in here what's wrong with me, and they all beat around the bush. One nurse says "What do you think is wrong?" and another tells me "Just be patient. Wait until the doctor arrives." Well, I'm tired of being patient. What's wrong with me?*

Expressed thoughts:

I want the truth from you. What's wrong with me?

Implied thoughts:

I wonder whether I'm seriously ill.

Mr. Wilson relates an experience to the nurse and openly expresses his impatience with the staff. Underneath that impatience is the more intense feeling of anger. Mr. Wilson is afraid that there is something seriously wrong with him and that this is why no one is being honest with him. His arguing is motivated by fears.

Recognizing Thoughts: Exercise 3

Read the following statement and distinguish between expressed and implied thoughts.

> *Sarah Turner: I'm so happy. My family's been so nice to me since I've been sick. My husband has been very thoughtful. He's come to visit me every day, and today he even sent me flowers.*

Expressed thoughts:

Implied thoughts:

Below are some possible statements of the expressed and implied thoughts contained in the patient's statement.

> **Sarah Turner: *I'm so happy. My family's been so nice to me since I've been sick. My husband's been very thoughtful. He's come to visit me every day, and today he even sent me flowers.***

Expressed thoughts:

> *My family's been so nice to me since I've been sick. My husband's been very thoughtful.*

Implied thoughts:

> *My family is usually more thoughtful than my husband. My husband usually isn't this nice. My husband affects how I feel.*

Clarifying Thoughts: Exercise 1

Read the following statements and identify the expressed and implied thoughts. Write a clarification response that attends to each patient's thoughts.

> ***Stan:***   *That was my sister Jo Ann who just left. I haven't seen her in years. She came all the way from Salt Lake City to visit me. I feel wonderful just seeing her again.*

Nurse's clarification of patient's thoughts:

> ***Clara:***   *I'm scared. I still can't see. The doctor said my loss of vision would be temporary. What's going on?*

Nurse's clarification of patient's thoughts:

Below are some possible clarification responses for the patients' statements presented.

> **Stan:** *That was my sister Jo Ann who just left. I haven't seen her in years. She came all the way from Salt Lake City to visit me. I feel wonderful just seeing her again.*

Nurse's clarification of patient's thoughts:

> *Your sister must really care about you to travel so far to visit you.*

Correct responses should focus on Jo Ann's concern for her brother. They may or may not focus on Stan's expressed feelings.

> **Clara:** *I'm scared. I still can't see. The doctor said my loss of vision would be temporary. What's going on?*

Nurse's clarification of patient's thoughts:

> *You're afraid that your loss of vision is a permanent one.*

Correct responses should reflect the patient's expressed feelings and focus on the patient's implied thoughts regarding the possible permanence of her condition.

Recognizing Thoughts and Feelings: Exercise 1

Read the following statement and identify the expressed and implied thoughts and feelings.

> ***Frank Rodgers: This food has no taste. I feed my dog better than this, and he doesn't pay me $120 a day for room and board! Just because I can't leave is no reason you should feed me this stuff.***

Expressed thoughts:

Expressed feelings:

Implied thoughts:

Implied feelings:

Below are some possible statements of the expressed and implied thoughts and feelings contained in Frank's message.

Frank Rodgers: *This food has no taste. I feed my dog better than this, and he doesn't pay me $120 a day for room and board! Just because I can't leave is no reason you should feed me this stuff.*

Expressed thoughts:

Just because I can't leave is no reason you should feed me this stuff.

Expressed feelings:

(None)

Implied thoughts:

I'm not getting my money's worth. You're taking advantage of me.

Implied feelings:

Anger, frustration, helplessness

Recognizing Thoughts and Feelings: Exercise 2

Consider the following statement. Distinguish between the patient's expressed and implied thoughts and feelings.

> *Barbara Bingham: I just ran into some friends of mine in the hall. When I invited them to come down to my room, they said they had to go. It seemed like they were here visiting someone else, but, since they didn't say who, I didn't ask. I wonder what's going on?*

Expressed thoughts:

Expressed feelings:

Implied thoughts:

Implied feelings:

Below are some possible statements of the expressed and implied thoughts and feelings contained in the patient's statement.

> **Barbara Bingham:** *I just ran into some friends of mine in the hall. When I invited them to come down to my room, they said they had to go. It seemed like they were here visiting someone else, but, since they didn't say who, I didn't ask. I wonder what's going on?*

Expressed thoughts:

It seemed like they were here visiting someone else.

Expressed feelings:

(None)

Implied thoughts:

They didn't want to see me. I wonder why? Who could they be visiting?

Implied feelings:

Confusion, rejection, hurt, disappointment

Clarifying Thoughts and Feelings: Exercise 1

Read the following patient statement. Underline the expressed thoughts and feelings and identify the implied thoughts and feelings. Write a clarification response that focuses on the significant thoughts and feelings, both expressed and implied.

> *Janet: I haven't had a visitor for days. Even my husband hasn't come to see me. I feel that you're the only person who cares what happens to me.*

Nurse's clarification of patient's thoughts and feelings:

Below are some possible clarifications of the patient's statement. Numerous clarifications are possible, but the most helpful responses will relate the patient's unexpressed thoughts and feelings.

> ***Janet:*** *I haven't had a visitor for days. Even my husband hasn't come to see me. I feel that you're the only person who cares what happens to me.*

Nurse's clarification of patient's thoughts and feelings:

1. *You're upset because your husband hasn't come to visit you.*
2. *You feel rejected by your husband.*
3. *You feel lonely because I'm the only person who demonstrates caring to you.*

Clarifying Thoughts and Feelings: Exercise 2

Read the following statement by the son of a patient. Underline the expressed thoughts and feelings and identify the implied thoughts and feelings. Write a clarification response that focuses on the significant thoughts and feelings, both expressed and implied.

> ***Joseph Thomas:*** ***She's dead. My mother. I can't believe it. It was just routine surgery. It shouldn't have happened. What are we going to do without her?***

Nurse's clarification of Joseph's thoughts and feelings:

Below are some possible clarifications of Joseph's statement. Numerous clarifications are possible, but the most helpful responses will relate the patient's unexpressed thoughts and feelings.

> **Joseph Thomas:** **She's dead. My mother. I can't believe it. It was just routine surgery. It shouldn't have happened. What are we going to do without her?**

Nurse's clarification of Joseph's thoughts and feelings:

1. *You're in a state of shock over your mother's death. You don't know how to deal with it.*
2. *You're upset because you think your mother's death was a mistake.*
3. *You think your mother's death shouldn't have happened—that it was the doctor's fault—and that's upsetting.*

RECOGNIZING HELPFUL RESPONSES

It is difficult to explain how one discriminates between potentially helpful and potentially unproductive clarification responses. It's even more difficult to detail the criteria used in determining the best of several clarification responses. The actual usefulness of a response can be determined only after it has been presented and the patient has given a reaction to it. However, there are a few basic guidelines for determining potential usefulness, and those will be outlined here.

First, a good clarification response *facilitates patient self-disclosure.* It should encourage the patient to express experiences, thoughts, and feelings more freely and communicate to the patient the nurse's interest in the problem. Clarification responses will prompt disclosure if they are neither too shallow nor too insightful. Responses that are too shallow are less meaningful than the patient's original statement. They communicate to the patient that the nurse is already frightened by the depth of the patient's communication. Shallow responses indirectly ask the patient to shift the conversation to safer ground. Responses that are too insightful cut through the patient's normal defenses. Highly insightful statements that are expressed too early in the relationship do not prompt disclosure; rather, they cause the patient to retreat and to disclose less than before.

Second, a good clarification response *communicates understanding.* It says to the patient, "I understand the experience you've told me about and the impact of that experience on you. I understand what you've shared with me and even some of that which you have only implied." A good clarification response proves to the speaker that you understand what is being said.

Third, a good response *attends to the patient's feelings.* It communicates a sensitivity to the patient's feelings about the situation and says "I understand the feelings you've shared with me and even some of the ones you've not yet chosen to share." It's important to encourage discussion of feelings because many patients' problems have their roots in the realm of emotions. Communication to a person that you both understand and accept his or her feelings is a very personal experience. Ignoring the feelings expressed is a rejection of that person's most private world.

Fourth, a good clarification response *attends* to the *thoughts that are related to the patient's feelings.* It communicates understanding not only of how the patient feels but also of why she or he feels that way. It relates the patient's implied and expressed feelings. It says "I understand that you feel this way because...."

Helpful Responding: Exercise 1

Read the following statement and select the clarification response that is most helpful.

Inez: *That physical therapist! When is she going to stop giving me the same exercises to do? It makes me mad. These exercises are a waste of my time.*

Mr. Dawson: A. *The physical therapist always gives you the same exercises to do. You'd rather have more difficult ones.*
B. *You're worried about physical therapy because you think the exercises the therapist gives you aren't going to help.*
C. *You're bored with physical therapy.*

If you picked A, turn to page 175.
If you picked B, turn to page 176.
If you picked C, turn to page 177.

You picked A

The physical therapist always gives you the same exercises to do. You'd rather have more difficult ones.

This is not the most helpful response. It reflects the speaker's experience and unexpressed thoughts and makes a guess at what the patient wants the physical therapist to do. A better response would include mention of the patient's feelings and her thoughts related to those feelings.

Inez's reaction to the response you selected would tell the nurse whether his assumption about more difficult exercises was correct. The patient might respond positively or she might suggest that she'd rather give up on the idea of physical therapy altogether. Guesses about what the patient wants to do about a situation are riskier and less helpful than clarifications of the patient's feelings about the situation.

Return to page 174 and try again.

You picked B

> *You're worried about physical therapy because you think the exercises the therapist gives you aren't going to help.*

Congratulations. This is the correct response. It elaborates both the patient's thoughts and her feelings. It assumes that the feeling underlying her anger is one of concern and that she is concerned because she doesn't think the exercises assigned by the therapist will remedy her condition. The response you selected brings this assumption into the open. The patient can either reject or accept this statement, but in either case she knows that she has been heard by the nurse. If Mr. Dawson's assumption is correct, Inez can now openly express her fear about the possible permanence of her injuries. Perhaps talking to the nurse and having him respond positively will encourage her to also discuss the problem with the physical therapist involved.

Turn to page 178.

You picked C

You're bored with physical therapy

This is not the most helpful response. It focuses only on the patient's feelings. It ignores both the experiential and the cognitive components of the message. The response attempts to focus on the patient's feelings but does so in a very shallow manner. Inez is feeling more than just bored, and this response might give her the idea that the nurse is bored with the conversation.

Return to page 174 and try again.

Helpful Responding: Exercise 2

Read the following statement and select the clarification response that is most helpful.

> **Anita Adams:** *I feel very distant from my family. I don't know what's wrong. All of a sudden I can't communicate with anyone. We were all so close before, and now when I'm talking to them, I feel like I'm talking to strangers.*
>
> **Mr. Tenley:** A. *It's hard for you to understand why you and your family aren't as close as you once were.*
> B. *You feel confused. You think maybe there's something wrong with you because you can't communicate with your family.*
> C. *You would like things to be better between you and your family.*

If you picked A, turn to page 179.
If you picked B, turn to page 180.
If you picked C, turn to page 181.

You picked A

It's hard for you to understand why you and your family aren't as close as you once were.

This is a great response, but it's not the best one. This response underlines Ms. Adams' confusion about what is happening to her relationship with her family. But Ms. Adams thinks she is responsible for the distance between her and her family: "I don't know what's wrong (with me)." A better response would demonstrate understanding of the patient's feelings of responsibility as well as the depth of her confusion.

Return to page 178 and try again to pick the best response.

You picked B

> *You feel confused. You think maybe there's something wrong with you because you can't communicate with your family.*

Congratulations. This was a difficult one, but you made the correct selection. This patient is troubled by her inability to maintain close relationships with the members of her family. Her references to herself indicate her feelings of personal responsibility for the problem: "I feel like I'm talking to strangers," "I can't communicate with anyone," "I don't know what's wrong." In her statement "I don't know what's wrong," "with me" is implied. This statement indicates that Anita is assuming responsibility for her difficulty with the family. She also believes that the problem is a recent one, as indicated by the phrases "all of a sudden" and "we were all so close before." The response you selected also attends to the patient's feeling of confusion—something the two other responses ignored.

Turn to page 182.

You picked C

You would like things to be better between you and your family.

This is not the best response. It focuses on the patient's desire that her relationship with her family would be better, which is implied by her original statement. However, of the implications made, this is the least important because it focuses on a solution rather than on the problem.

Return to page 178 and try again to pick the best response.

CHARACTERISTICS OF CLARIFICATION

1. Clarification responses are usually stated in the second person; that is, they refer to the patient rather than to the nurse.
2. Common stems that begin clarification responses are:
   a. "You seem to feel that..."
   b. "You seem to think that..."
   c. "It sounds to me like you..."
   d. "Underneath it all, you really..."
3. The clarification response is based on the internal frame of reference of the patient. The nurse tries to understand the patient as if he or she were the patient.
4. The nurses may respond to any combination of the component parts of the speaker's message. The listener may respond to the content, the feelings, or both.
5. The clarification response amplifies the meaning of the original statement. It is an attempt to add clarity to the patient's message.
6. The clarifying listener is in tune with the patient's expressed feelings and thoughts as well as his or her implied feelings and thoughts.
7. The clarifying listener amplifies the thoughts and feelings of the speaker. The listener shares with the speaker his or her perceptions of the patient's unexpressed thoughts and feelings.

CONSEQUENCES OF CLARIFICATION RESPONSES

Because of the more sensitive listening that clarification provides, the patient's behavior should show some changes. Some changes will be similar to those induced by reflective listening. A clarifying listener is *encouraging to the speaker* and indicates to the speaker that the nurse is *listening very carefully.* The patient is reinforced by this close attention and usually will express himself or herself in greater depth thereafter.

The patient will realize that his or her *communication is not always as clear and complete as she or he thought,* since at times what the nurse heard and what the patient thought was said were not the same.

The clarifying listener tries to hear what the patient leaves unsaid as well as what is said. By focusing the attention of the interaction on these unexpressed areas, the nurse facilitates patient elaboration and exploration of them. Thus, *clarification promotes a more thorough definition of the problem* in addition to increased patient self-disclosure.

A clarifying listener attempts to state the patient's feelings in a clearer manner than the patient is able to do. The nurse tries to indicate to the patient that he or she understands even what the patient finds difficult to express clearly. An obvious result of clarification, then, is that the *patient gains a better understanding of himself or herself,* which might later prove useful in problem resolution.

The clarifying listener amplifies the patient's thoughts and feelings. The patient will at times verify these clarifications and at times refute them. The nurse will come to *realize that his or her assumptions aren't always as accurate as she or he thought.*

Finally, both the *patient and the nurse will become more satisfied with their conversations.* Instead of two people casually listening to each other, a conversational flow is established wherein one person is really trying to understand the thoughts and feelings of another.

CLASSIFICATION EXERCISE

Read the following statements and circle the letter that indicates to which type of response the statement applies.

R = Reflection
C = Clarification
B = Both reflection and clarification
N = Neither reflection nor clarification

R C B N   1. Focuses on the speaker

R C B N   2. Amplifies

R C B N   3. Offers solutions

R C B N   4. Acknowledges the problem

R C B N   5. States underlying feelings

R C B N   6. Defines the problem more clearly

R C B N   7. Asks questions

R C B N   8. Uses nonverbal clues

R C B N   9. May restate any information imparted by the speaker

R C B N   10. Is interchangeable with original message.

R C B N   11. Makes assumptions

R C B N   12. Evaluates the speaker

R C B N   13. Focuses on implied thoughts and feelings

R C B N   14. Increases self-disclosure

R C B N   15. Focuses on the listener's experiences

The classification exercise on the previous page summarizes the major characteristics of reflective and clarification responses. Check your answers with those listed here and evaluate your performance as indicated below.

1. Both

2. Clarification

3. Neither

4. Both

5. Clarification

6. Both

7. Neither

8. Both

9. Both

10. Reflection

11. Clarification

12. Neither

13. Clarification

14. Both

15. Neither

13-15 correct = Excellent. Go on to the next chapter.
10-12 correct = Good. Go on to the next chapter.
Less than 10 correct = You need to review Chapter 6.

7
Questioning

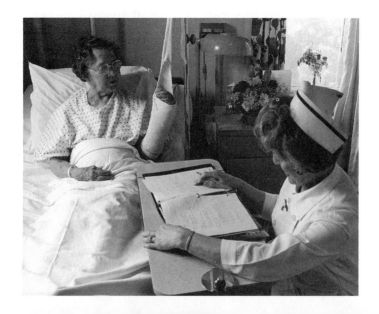

Questions constitute a large part of human interaction. Despite the risks inherent in their use, they can facilitate nurse-patient interactions by inviting the patient to speak, saving time, making general concepts more specific, and combining specific examples into general themes. Questions can assist the nurse in sorting out the information the patient provides. Questions can even facilitate a warm, trusting climate in which two partners work together to reach mutually agreed upon goals.

Questioning is not without liabilities, however. Questioning has often been greatly misused and overused by nurses. When misuse occurs, it is damaging to the nurse-patient relationship. Several writers (Gazda et al., 1982; Patterson, 1985) have commented on the negative effects of misused questions. The two biggest misuses are related to the quantity and quality of questions.

INAPPROPRIATE QUANTITY OF QUESTIONS

All too frequently, nurses rely on questioning to carry the weight of the interview. Questions are an efficient way to get at specific information but they often inhibit a free flow of information, which is essential for problem resolution. The nurse has the ultimate responsibility for structuring the interaction: however, the responsibility for self-disclosure, self-exploration, and the ultimate decision making rests with the patient. The nurse is only responsible for facilitating these objectives.

Many reasons can be offered to explain the overuse of questioning by nurses. One is the haste with which basic information is obtained from the patient. Many nurses believe that asking direct questions is the quickest way to obtain information. Another explanation is the lack of basic understanding of how to use other response styles to effectively facilitate disclosure. In other cases, the nurse simply does not know what the patient is saying.

When too many questions are asked, many of them are probably inappropriate. Excessive questioning places the patient in a dependent role, thereby reducing self-exploration. Excessive questioning also places responsibility for problem solving on the nurses and often generates feelings of defensiveness, hostility, and resentment on the part of the patient.

INAPPROPRIATE QUALITY OF QUESTIONS

Certain questions, by their very nature, are generally considered ineffective for facilitative communication

"Why" questions.   Nurses should generally avoid "why" questions. Only occasionally do they serve a useful purpose. "Why" questions have considerable underlying implications that the nurse may not have intended. Often they seem like an accusation since they require an explanation or justification by the patient. They immediately put the patient on the defensive.

A "why" question is asked to determine causality, motivation, or intent. The questions also convey value judgments. Implicit in a "why" question is the suggestion that what the patient did or said was wrong, bad, or inappropriate. For example, "Why did you take aspirin?" suggests that aspirin was not the correct medication.

Obviously, the utility of "why" questions is doubtful and their effect counterproductive. They fail to communicate the facilitative condition of respect to the patient, since they require justification.

Most questions that use "why" can be rephrased into a more facilitative form by using the words *how* or *what.* Questions phrased in this manner require the patient to relate or describe the situation. There is no inherent causality or motivation associated with the answer.

Example 1

Why: Why are you so depressed today?

Better: What happened today?

Example 2

Why: Why didn't you bring this baby in sooner?

Better: What did you do when you first noticed this rash?

Example 3

Why: Why do you come to the nurses' office five times a day?

Better: How does coming to the nurses' office make you feel better?

Rephrasing "why" questions to other forms will help the patient be more open and assist the nurse in obtaining the information needed. By carefully considering the reason and purpose for each question, it will be easy to ask the most appropriate question in the most appropriate manner.

Multiple-choice questions.   Multiple-choice questions occur when the nurse gives the patient a question and several alternative answers.

Example 1:   Did you take tylenol or aspirin?

Example 2:   Are you worried about your husband's reaction or your daughter's?

Multiple-choice questions tend to bias the patient's answer. It is better to delete the multiple-choice alternatives and simply ask the question. This way, the patient will answer in his or her own words and you will get a more accurate response.

Example 1:   What did you take for the pain?

Example 2:   What are you worried about?

Multiple questions.   Multiple questions occur when the nurse poses several questions all at the same time to the patient. The questions may differ in quality and importance. The most common response in this situation is to select one of the questions and answer it. Usually the patient will answer by responding to the least threatening question. Multiple questions can be confusing to both the patient and the nurse.

Example: Would you like to go home tomorrow? Are your stitches still sore? Do you have to walk up stairs to get to your house?

Some of these questions would be useful if taken alone, but when they are asked simultaneously, they leave the patient in a quandary over which to answer first.

A nurse who tries to solve a problem too soon or fears that he or she may forget to ask a particular question will often use this form of questioning. One question at a time is the obvious remedy.

Rhetorical questions.   Rhetorical questions are not really questions. They don't require an answer and, in many cases, have no answer. They are a way for the nurse to state a given belief or emotion in the form of a question.

Example 1:   What am I supposed to do with you?

Example 2:   Why does everybody get sick at 3:00 in the morning?

Questions of this type do little to further information gathering or patient self-exploration. Rhetorical questions are loaded with value judgments that become irritating to the patient. They communicate neither understanding nor respect and should be avoided.

Accusative questions.   The purpose of an accusative question is to accuse the patient of specific acts rather than to seek information or facilitate self-exploration.

Example: You didn't take your medicine, did you?

Example: Are you coming to my office just to get out of the gym?

Accusations of this type leave the patient with no recourse but defensiveness or counterhostility. Questions of this type communicate understanding or respect. They are, by their very nature, highly threatening and have no useful function. Accusative questions should be avoided.

APPROPRIATE QUESTIONING

Facilitative questions communicate an interest in the patient and his or her communication. Facilitative questions are sensitive to the thoughts and feelings of the patient, and are directly related to the patient's problem. In contrast, nonfacilitative questions are ineffective because they (1) redirect the focus of the conversation to an irrelevant issue by changing the subject, (2) are overly threatening in their purpose, and (3) demonstrate a lack of understanding to the patient. The nonfacilitative questioner becomes an interrogator, assuming an aggressive role that will endanger any relationship that has been established so far. Discrimination between appropriate and inappropriate questions become a critical and necessary skill for nurses to master. It is also important for the nurse to understand what types of questions produce what types of responses.

OPEN VERSUS CLOSED QUESTIONS

All questions can be classified as either open or closed. Closed questions require only a brief factual response or a yes or no answer. They limit the number of possible responses and do not encourage the speaker to talk. The most likely response to a closed question is a one- or two-word answer. The patient then waits for the next question. Here are some examples of closed questions.

Example 1:   What type of medication are you taking?

Example 2:   How long have you been having headaches?

Example 3:   Do you want to try getting up?

All three of these questions limit the patient's response. The first requires the name of a medicine, the second a time, and the third a simple yes or no. Closed questions are helpful when taking a patient's history or soliciting very specific information, but in most other situations they limit the free flow of information.

On the other hand, open-ended questions prompt the speaker to reveal more information. The number of possible responses to an open-ended question is unlimited. It allows the patient a freedom of response that is impossible with a closed question. Although the response to an open-ended question will most likely be longer than a response to a closed question, it is also likely that the patient will wait for the next question after completing his or her response. Since a series of questions always establishes the nurse as the "master of ceremonies" no matter what types of questions are used, questions should be used sparingly. Look at the following examples of open questions and notice that the responses available to the client are limitless.

Example 1: How was your baby acting last night?

Example 2: Explain the advantages you see for leaving the hospital.

Study the following stimulus statements and and nurse responses. Notice the difference between open and closed responses as they apply to the same patient statement.

High School Student: Steve is into drugs. He really doesn't have his head on straight. I don't know what to do.

School Nurse (closed questions)
1. Which Steve?
2. Has Steve ever dropped acid?

School Nurse (open questions)
1. What does Steve do that tells you he's having problems?
2. How does Steve's being into drugs affect you?

The key difference between open and closed questions lies in the structure of the questions. Open questions allow a wide variety of responses. Closed questions limit the patient's responses. Because of this difference, they also differ in their communication of respect. Open questions communicate respect to the patient. They communicate acceptance of the patient as a person and demonstrate, within limits, what is appropriate and what is inappropriate to the problem. They further demonstrate respect by allowing the patient to talk about the problem in his or her own words. Closed questions, on the other hand, have the tendency to evoke counterproductive feelings of defensiveness, hostility, and frustration. Additionally, they negate further patient self-exploration by bringing the discussion to a close.

Here is an example of the use of closed questions in trying to begin a dialogue with a patient.

Mrs. Ricardo: Hi, Bob. You wanted to see me?

Bob: I guess so.

Mrs. Ricardo: What's the matter ?

Bob: My mother wants to transfer me to another hospital.

Mrs. Ricardo: Is she serious?

Bob: Yes.

Mrs. Ricardo: Is this something she's been thinking about for a while?

Bob: I don't know. She just told me today.

Here is an example of how open questions could be used in the same interview.

Mrs. Ricardo: Hi, Bob. Did you ask to see me?

Bob: Yes I did.

Mrs. Ricardo: Tell me, what's on your mind?

Bob: My mother wants to transfer me to another hospital.

Mrs. Ricardo: What were the reasons your mother gave you?

Bob: She said that this hospital is too far from our house. Now that I am getting better she wants me at a hospital nearer home.

In this example, the open-ended question facilitates further discussion and exploration, whereas the closed questions require more questions, thus leading to an interrogation. Ideally, the nurse's questions should be designed to facilitate clarification of what has been said. They should allow the patient the freedom to share the problem in his or her own words.

Open versus Closed Questioning: Exercise 1

Given the following statement by a patient to a nurse, which of the following nurse statements is open-ended?

> *Mrs. Chang: Things aren't right. All these drugs are making me forgetful. Today I left my purse at a store.*

> *Nurse Responses: A. How much money was missing?*
> *B. Did you ever have a day like this before?*
> *C. What are some of the other symptoms you are having?*

If you picked A, go to page 196.
If you picked B, go to page 197.
If you picked C, go to page 198.

You picked A

How much money was missing?

You were to pick the example of an open-ended question. This is not it. This is a closed question since the range of possible responses is greatly limited. Mrs. Chang should respond to this question by citing an amount of money. This question does not require that the patient reveal relevant information about herself. Most likely, the patient will respond by stating an amount and then waiting for the next question.

An open-ended question would encourage Mrs. Chang to reveal more information. The range of possible responses would not be limited to a particular set. Freedom of response is the difference between open and closed questions. Questions that require yes or no answers are examples of closed questions.

*Return to page 195 and
pick out the open question.*

You picked B

Did you ever have a day like this before?

You were to pick an example of an open-ended question. This is not it. This is a closed question since the range of possible responses is greatly limited. It requires only a yes or no answer. At most, Mrs. Chang could respond, "Yes, way back in November I had a day that was almost as bad."

An open-ended question would encourage Mrs. Chang to reveal more information. The range of possible responses would not be limited to a particular set. An open-ended question usually does not solicit short, concise answers. The key difference between open and closed questions is the freedom of response allowed. If there is only one correct response or if the number of responses is greatly limited, the question is closed.

Return to page 195, and pick out the open question.

You picked C

What are some of the other symptoms you are having?

This is an open question. There is no predefined list of responses from which Mrs. Chang must choose. She is free to describe her symptoms in as much or as little detail as she likes. This question encourages the patient to reveal more information about her symptoms.

The other alternatives limit Mrs. Chang in the type of response she is free to make. Question A calls for an amount of money. Question B requires a yes or no answer. Both of these questions put limits on the type and length of the patient's responses.

Think of questions as test questions. Multiple choice, true or false, and matching are all examples of closed questions. The student has a limited number of responses from which to choose. Arithmetic problems, where the student is expected to add, subtract, multiply, or divide pairs of numbers, are closed questions since there is only one acceptable response. Essay questions are open questions, since freedom of response and the number of acceptable responses is diverse.

Turn to page 199.

Open versus Closed Questioning: Exercise 2

Read the following statement by a student to the school nurse. Which of the following nurse responses is a closed question?

Marc: *I've had to share a room with my kid brother ever since he was born. My sister gets to have a room all to herself. I'm being treated unfairly again—as usual.*

Nurse Responses: A. *In what other situations do you think your parents treat you unfairly?*
B. *How many sisters do you have?*
C. *Why do you feel so mistreated at home?*

If you picked A, turn to page 200.
If you picked B, turn to page 201.
If you picked C, turn to page 202.

You picked A

In what other situations do you think your parents treat you unfairly?

You were to pick the example of a closed question. This is not it. The above question is an open-ended question. An open-ended question allows the speaker a greater range of acceptable responses. In response to the above question, Marc could describe one or several incidents in as much or as little detail as he chooses.

In response to a closed question the speaker must respond from a predetermined list of acceptable answers. Yes or no questions are closed questions. Closed questions inhibit interactions, since the speaker merely answers the question and then waits for the next question to be directed to him.

Return to page 199 and pick out the closed question.

You picked B

How many sisters do you have?

You picked the correct response. This is a closed question. It limits the type of response in that there is only one correct answer. Marc's response to the question will be to say a number and then wait for the next question. Obviously, this type of question will not encourage Marc to talk openly about himself.

The two alternative questions—"In what other situations do you think your parents treat you unfairly?" and "Why do you feel so mistreated at home?"—allow for more extended responses and a greater freedom of response style.

Turn to page 203.

You picked C

Why do you feel so mistreated at home?

You were to pick an example of a closed question. This is not it. This is an open question that allows Marc a range of acceptable responses. In response to this question, Marc could describe why he feels mistreated at home as well as his reaction to the situation. This question does not greatly limit the nature or the length of the response.

Closed questions limit the freedom of expression of the responder and limit the length of the acceptable response. A closed question would inhibit interaction, since Marc would merely answer the question and then wait for the next question to be directed to him. Even questions that allow a greater range of acceptable responses can be poor questions. The above "why" question could threaten the patient and close down his desire to respond at all.

Return to page 199 and pick out the closed question.

Open versus Closed Questioning: Exercise 3

Many closed questions can be rewritten as open questions. Rewrite the following closed questions as open questions.

> **Mrs. Harrington:** **I'm scared. I'm afraid I'm going to have a miscarriage. I've got to have this baby. I've just got to.**

Closed question:

Have you ever had a miscarriage before?

Open question:

Closed question:

Is there a special reason you have to have this baby?

Open question:

Following are possible open-ended responses.

Mrs. Harrington: *I'm scared. I'm afraid I'm going to have a miscarriage. I've got to have this baby. I've just got to.*

Closed question:

Have you ever had a miscarriage before?

Open question:

Describe the previous problems you've had while pregnant.

Closed question:

Is there any special reason you have to have this baby?

Open question:

What are the reasons you have to have this baby?

Open versus Closed Questioning: Exercise 4

Rewrite the following closed questions as open questions.

> **Mr. Miller:** *I saw you in there with all the other nurses. Were you talking about me? I know I'm the problem. I don't mean to be. It's just that I hate it here.*

Closed question:

Is the food the reason you hate it here?

Open question:

Closed question:

Would you rather be home?

Open question:

Here are some sample open questions.

Mr. Miller: *I saw you in there with all the other nurses. Were you talking about me? I know I'm the problem. I don't mean to be. I just hate it here.*

Closed question:

Is the food the reason you hate it here?

Open question:

What don't you like about the hospital?

Closed question:

Would you rather be home?

Open question:

Describe where you would rather be.

QUESTION ORIENTATION

Before formulating a question, the nurse must decide to what aspect of the answer to respond. The nurse has a choice of responding to the experience the speaker presents, to his or her thoughts about the experience, to his or her feelings about the experience, or to any combination of the three.

A facilitative question is directed at material already mentioned by the speaker, as opposed to being directed at new or tangential information. Facilitative questions related to the experiences already expressed by the speaker are often termed *experientially related questions*. They attempt to get the speaker to supply missing information and increase the listener's understanding of the material. Cognitively oriented questions explore significant thoughts more deeply. Affectively oriented questions are directed at feelings already mentioned by the speaker. A facilitative question may also ask the speaker to define feelings thus far only implied. Most messages contain two or three components. The speaker must decide which of these to address.

Let's look at an example:

Nancy: My son's really sick. They want me to leave him here until the end of the week for tests. I don't know if I can live without him. I'm scared.

The nurse can formulate an experientially oriented question designed to obtain more information, "What is wrong with your son?" or a cognitively oriented question designed to clarify thoughts, "How do you feel about leaving your son here for a week?" or an affectively oriented question, "What are you afraid of?"

Question Orientation: Exercise 1

Read this stimulus statement and formulate the following open questions.

> ***Joan:*** ***I'm so mad at that doctor! He didn't show up this morning to sign my discharge papers. I want to be home by the weekend.***

Experientially oriented question:

Cognitively oriented question:

Affectively oriented question:

Here are some possible answers.

> **Joan:** I'm so mad at that doctor. He didn't show up this morning to sign my discharge papers. I want to be home by the weekend.

Experientially oriented question:

What gave you the impression that the doctor was going to discharge you this morning?

Cognitively oriented question:

What is the reason you want to be home by the weekend?

Affectively oriented question:

What other feelings do you have?

Question Orientation: Exercise 2

Read the following stimulus statement and formulate the following closed questions.

> **Carol:** *I haven't had a visitor for days. Even my husband hasn't come to see me! I feel you're the only person that cares what happens to me.*

Experientially oriented question:

Cognitively oriented question:

Affectively oriented question:

Here are some possible closed questions.

Carol: *I haven't had a visitor for days. Even my husband hasn't come to see me! I feel you're the only person who cares what happens to me.*

Experientially oriented question:

When did you have your last visitor?

Cognitively oriented question:

Do you think your husband is too busy at work?

Affectively oriented question:

Do you feel rejected?

FACILITATIVE QUESTIONING

A facilitative question shows the patient that the nurse is actively listening. It conveys understanding and should be directly relevant to the patient's problem. A facilitative question is asked for a specific purpose and adds meaning to the nurse-patient interaction process. It is an open-ended question related to either the content or feelings of the message. It is also related to information already discussed by the patient and highlights the major problem at hand. A good facilitative question solicits missing information or clarifies previously encountered material. It can help start an interview or clarify patient behavior. A facilitative question communicates understanding and respect. Most importantly, it helps the patient understand himself or herself.

Facilitative Questioning: Exercise 1

Which of the following nurse questions is the most helpful?

> *Harry:* I'm really depressed about the ways things are going on between me and one of the other patients on this ward. It's never been like this before. We don't get along at all. It seems like the least little thing just gets us going at each other.

> *Nurse Responses:* A. *How do you get along with the other patients?*
> B. *What patient are you having trouble with?*
> C. *What types of things get you "going at each other"?*

If you picked A, turn to page 214.
If you picked B, turn to page 215.
If you picked C, turn to page 216.

You picked A

How do you get along with the other patients?

You were to choose the most helpful question. This is not it. This question shifts attention away from the major problem at hand to a secondary issue. This patient is concerned about his relationship with a particular patient. Drawing his attention away from this issue to his relationship with the other patients serves no purpose at this time. This question refers to neither previously mentioned content or previously mentioned feelings.

This question does have two good points: it is open and it actively seeks more information.

Turn back one page and try again.

You picked B

What patient are you having trouble with?

You were to pick out the example of the most helpful question. This is not it. Although this question seeks more information about the problem at hand, it is not the most helpful. This is a closed question and the information it seeks is of trivial importance.

*Turn back two pages
and try again.*

You picked C

What types of things get you "going at each other"?

You chose the correct response. This is the most helpful question. It seeks specific information about why this patient is having trouble with another patient. It is open ended and, therefore, allows a great deal of freedom in the response. It is directly related to the content the patient already described. It seeks clarification of the sentence, "It seems like the least little thing just gets us going at each other." It asks, in a sense, "Namely, what little things?"

Turn to the next page.

Facilitative Questioning: Exercise 2

Given the following patient statements, which of the following nurse responses is the most helpful?

> *Allison:* *My brother called last night. The one that's in the Army. He's not going to be able to come to see me. They won't give him time off. He has to leave for Germany tomorrow. I won't be able to see him for a year. I really wanted him to see the baby before he leaves. We've always been so close.*
>
> *Nurse Responses:* A. *Do you have any other brothers in the Army?*
> B. *How do you feel, knowing he's not going to be able to come?*
> C. *Why don't you send him a picture of the baby?*

If you picked A, turn to page 218.
If you picked B, turn to page 219.
If you picked C, turn to page 220.

You picked A

Do you have any other brothers in the Army?

You were suppose to choose the most helpful question. This is not it. This question is irrelevant to the problem at hand. This patient misses her brother who is in the Army. It does not matter whether this is her only brother or if she has 10 other brothers in the Army. The fact is that Allison misses this brother, and wants him to see the baby before leaving for Germany.

Turn back one page and try again.

You picked B

How do you feel, knowing he's not going to be able to come?

Of the three options, this is the most helpful question. First, it is an open-ended question. The patient is given a great deal of freedom to express herself.

Second, it is related to feelings. It seeks expression of the implied feelings of hurt and disappointment. Allison has a lot of strong feelings about her brother leaving for Germany and not being able to see the baby before he goes. She did not express these feelings. This statement gives her the opportunity to do so.

Turn to page 221.

You picked C

Why don't you send him a picture of the baby?

You were to pick the most helpful question. This is not it. This question suggests a solution to one of the problems presented. However, it ignores the more important problem—that the patient will not be able to see her brother for a year.

Suggesting a solution to either problem at this point is premature. First, the nurse should help Allison more fully express the problem and her feelings related to it. Solutions such as the one suggested might prove helpful later.

*Turn to page 217
and try again.*

Facilitative Questioning: Exercise 3

Read the stimulus statement. Which of the following counselor questions is most helpful to this high school student?

William: Ted doesn't have his head on straight. He's into drugs. I can't relate to him at all anymore. I thought maybe you could talk to him.

Nurse Responses: A. *What type of drugs is Ted into?*
B. *In what ways are you having trouble relating to Ted?*
C. *Is Ted having trouble with his school work because of this problem?*

If you picked A, turn to page 222.
If you picked B, turn to page 223.
If you picked C, turn to page 224.

You picked A

What type of drug is Ted into?

You were to choose the most helpful question. This is not it. This is a closed question since the number of possible responses is limited. It seeks clarification of the term *drugs*. Knowing what kind of drugs Ted is taking might prove helpful to Ted, but in order to help William, the nurse should initially focus on the problem presented. A more helpful question would facilitate interaction by providing the opportunity for a diverse number of responses.

*Go back to page 221
and select another response.*

You picked B

In what ways are you having trouble relating to Ted?

This is a content-related question which seeks clarification of the phrase, "I can't relate to him at all any more." The nurse is soliciting specific examples of how William is having trouble relating to Ted.

This question is the most helpful since it focuses on William's relationship with Ted rather than on Ted and his drug problem. The question communicates to the speaker, "I am interested in you and your concerns."

Turn to page 226.

You picked C

Is Ted having trouble with his school work because of this problem?

You were to select the most helpful question. This is not it. This is a closed question. It requires a yes or no answer. It asks William to nullify or confirm the nurse's projections regarding the problem. The nurse is guessing that Ted's problem with drugs is affecting his school work. She is asking William if this is true rather than allowing him to express the problem himself.

This question steers William away from the major problem expressed. The relevancy of this question depends on whether or not Ted is having a problem with his school work. Instead of guessing at likely problems, the nurse should try to get William to clarify the problem already expressed.

Go back to page 221 and try again.

SUMMARY

Counseling is a verbal and nonverbal interaction process that includes the following basic objectives: (1) developing and maintaining a facilitative relationship, (2) facilitating patient self-exploration and self-understanding, and (3) working toward mutually agreed upon goals.

Facilitative questions—as well as the other verbal interaction skills of reflection, clarification, and summarization—can help the nurse achieve the basic objectives in the counseling process. The effective use of questions can contribute to the core conditions of empathic understanding, respect, and genuineness.

Nonfacilitative questions generally prove ineffective because they: (1) change the focus of the discussion to irrelevant issues, (2) are closed and do not allow the patient freedom of expression, (3) are overly threatening, and (4) demonstrate a lack of understanding of the patient.

Questions may be directed toward any of the three components of a patient's message—experiential, affective, or cognitive. The effective helper should direct his or her questioning to the most relevant component(s).

Appropriate questioning is an important adjunct to the nurse's verbal and nonverbal repertoire.

8
Focusing on Solutions

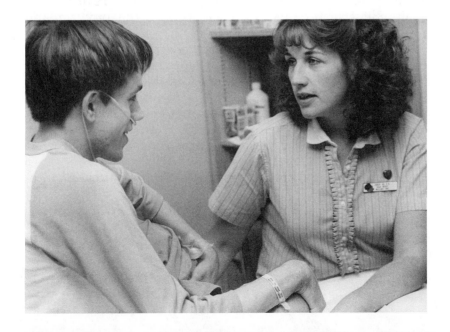

Reflective responses develop trust and facilitate patient disclosure by communicating understanding. Clarification responses expand the patient's statements, deepen the relationship between patient and nurse, and more clearly define the problem. Once the problem has been expressed and clearly defined, it's time to move on to the solution phase of the interaction. In this phase, alternatives are outlined and evaluated and a decision is made about what action is to be taken. The purpose of solution-oriented responses is to aid in this decision-making process. Solution-oriented responses communicate to the patient "I have listened to and understood what you've tried to express; now let's focus on what might be done about the situation."

In discussing solution-oriented responses, it is assumed that the patient has presented a problem to the nurse. If no problem has been presented, of course, then solution-oriented responses would not be appropriate. Also, many problems have no solution; in these cases, too, solution-oriented responses are inappropriate. In these two circumstances, the patient need only express himself or herself fully and know that the nurse is listening with understanding and respect.

Solution-oriented responses are not appropriate at the beginning of a conversation, when a patient is presenting a problem. The problem must be presented and explored in detail before solutions are considered. Talking about solutions before the problem has been carefully examined would be premature. The relevant aspects of the problem must be brought out first so that the solution will be a realistic and comprehensive response to all aspects of the problem and thus have a better chance for success.

A distinction must be made between solution-oriented responses and advice giving. Solution-oriented responses help the patient to consider the various possible solutions, rather than insist that the patient behave in a particular manner. They take the forms of suggestions, not commands. Solution-oriented responses focus on the patient and what she or he might do about the problem, not on someone else and what that person would do in the patient's situation.

Consider the following responses to this patient's statement.

John Nava: I want to leave here and get back to work. I'm sick of it here. I can't wait to get out of the hospital, but the doctor says I have to have more tests.

Mr. Young: A. You must not leave yet.

B. If I were you, I'd stay here and get the test done before going back to work.

C. There comes a time when most patients don't like the hospital very much, but they stick it out—and you should, too.

The first response is an example of advice giving. It tells the patient what to do. Such a response shows a lack of respect for the patient as a person who can decide for himself what he should do. Solution-oriented responses should indicate to the patient that the nurse believes the patient is capable of deciding what should be done.

In the second response, the nurse tells the patient what he would do if he were in John's place. What Mr. Young meant by his statement was that, if he were in a similar situation, he would not leave the hospital. But it is John who has the problem, and it is he who must decide what is best for him to do.

The third response tells the patient that other patients feel the same way about the hospital. The nurse continues by telling John that he should do what other patients have done—"stick it out." This statement ignores the fact that John is a unique individual with his own perceptions, needs, and goals. The way other patients have dealt with the problem may not be the right way for John.

Although all of these responses focus on what the patient should do, none of them is very helpful. Good solution-oriented responses help the patient to work through the problem-solving process. They help the patient decide what he or she wants to do. Solution-oriented responses usually fit into one of four types: (1) those that help the patient to shift discussion from exploration of the problem to consideration of possible solutions, (2) those that help the patient consider various specific solutions, (3) those that help the patient evaluate each solution, and (4) those that help the patient select a plan of action.

The following is an example of a patient's statement, followed by four possible responses. Each response demonstrates one of the four types of solution-oriented responses.

Mike Robinson: My history teacher was in today. She says she'll give me only a week to make up the report I missed, but I can't do it this week. I can't even get out of bed, so how am I supposed to get to the library to do the research? Besides, I have to get to bed so early here at the hospital—there's no way I can get that report done this week.

Ms. Rodriguez: A. Let's consider some things you could do.
B. Have you thought about trying to arrange for your Mom to bring in the library books?
C. What do you think would happen if you talked to your history teacher and asked for an extension?
D. Now that the alternatives are outlined, what are you going to do?

Response A helps the patient move from describing the problem to considering possible solutions. This is an example of the first type of solution-oriented response. No solution is suggested; the nurse only suggests that it might be appropriate to consider some solutions.

The second response encourages the patient to consider a specific solution. Responses of this type either offer solutions or encourage the patient to think of solutions for himself or herself. The nurse should always be aware that the patient may have thought of one or more possible solutions prior to talking with the nurse or during the course of their discussion. The patient should be encouraged to verbalize these solutions. The nurse may suggest any possible solutions that occur to him or her during the discussion or draw on his or her own personal experience or the experience of others who were in a similar situation. (Remember, however, that the focus should always remain on the patient.) In talking, the patient and nurse may mutually arrive at possible solutions. Finally, other people—such as friends, parents, relatives, teachers, or other members of the hospital staff—may have suggested possible solutions.

The third response encourages the speaker to consider the advantages and the disadvantages of a particular situation. The nurse's response asks Mike to consider what might have happened if he were to follow a particular plan of action—that is, talk to his history teacher again.

The fourth response asks the patient "What are you going to do now?" It invites him to look over the advantages and disadvantages of each alternative and made a decision. The sequence in which these solution-oriented responses are presented is the order in which they are most likely to be used during the discussion with a patient. After encouraging the patient to describe the situation, the nurse helps the patient to shift the focus to possible solutions, then to consider various specific solutions, then to evaluate those solutions, and finally to decide on a plan of action.

SHIFTING THE FOCUS

After the patient has fully explored and defined the problem, it's time to move on to the first phase of the solution-oriented process. The intention of this first phase is to shift the focus from the problem to its possible solutions. This might occur as quickly as 10 minutes after the initial problem is expressed or as long as 2 or 3 hours after the initial expression of the problem; in some cases it may not occur at all. Many problems presented by patients never reach the solution stage because some problems do not have solutions. Such problems are usually expressed not in hope of finding answers but for the satisfaction of being heard and understood.

It is important to stress that a shift to this stage of helping should occur only after the patient has fully explored the problem. It's better to err in the direction of too thoroughly defining the problem than to attempt to reach solutions prematurely. The correct time to shift the focus of discussion will be evident from the repetitious thoughts and feelings being expressed by the patient. If you attempt to shift from problem definition to solution finding and the patient ignores your response or tries to redefine the problem, then your solution-finding occurred too soon. Follow the patient's lead and more clearly explore and define the problem. Shift to the solution-finding process at a later time.

The purpose of a solution-oriented response is to shift the focus of helping from problem exploration and definition to solution finding, but the effects of this kind of response are far-reaching. The solution-oriented response asks the patient "What can you do about this problem?" This kind of response puts the responsibility on the patient to solve his or her own problem; it doesn't give the nurse the responsibility to solve the problem. It indicates respect for the patient as an independent person with the ability to solve the problem on his or her own. Solution-oriented responses should not foster dependence; rather, they should encourage the patient to solve the problem.

After the patient has suggested as many solutions as possible, it's time to move to the second phase of the solution process, which is the consideration of specific suggestions by the nurse. This may occur after the patient has suggested two solutions or twenty, but it always occurs after the patient has exhausted his or her list of suggestions. This second phase of the solution process, the nurse's suggestions, can sometimes lead the patient to formulate additional solutions, but it need not necessarily do so.

Shifting Focus: Exercise 1

Which of the following responses is an example of a solu-tion-oriented response that shifts the focus from exploration of the problem to possible solution?

Rachel Patterson: **As I said, I don't know what to do about physical therapy. I don't want to stop going, but it doesn't seem to be doing any good.**

Ms. Olsen: A. **Come with me and we'll tell the head nurse about this.**

B. **Why don't you see if you can work with a different therapist tomorrow?**

C. **Do you have any ideas about what you might do about this situation?**

If you picked A, turn to page 234.
If you picked B, turn to page 235.
If you picked C, turn to page 236.

You picked A

Come with me and we'll tell the head nurse about this.

This is an example not of shifting the focus but of a nurse telling the patient what to do. This response is in the form of a command, rather than a suggestion, and therefore is not a good solution-oriented response.

Had this response been phrased instead as "Do you think it would help if you told the head nurse?" it would have been a good example of a solution-oriented response, helping Rachel to consider specific solutions. (Notice that, when rephrased, it is presented as a suggestion for consideration, not as a command.) However, even this kind of response would be premature. It is important to first help the patient to express all of his or her own ideas about solutions to the problem; only then should the nurse begin to suggest solutions.

Return to page 233 and try again.

You picked B

Why don't you see if you can work with a different therapist tomorrow?

This is not the correct response. It is a solution-oriented response and is phrased as a suggestion, but it offers a specific solution, rather than helping to shift the focus from exploration of the problem to consideration of possible solutions. The first phase of the solution-oriented stage of helping is facilitating the suggestion of solutions by the patient. Only after the patient has exhausted his or her supply of possible solutions should the second phase of the process begin. In the second phase the nurse would make suggestions similar to that of response B.

Suggestions like that in response C will prompt further patient suggestions, and the process will continue. When as many solutions as possible have been suggested, the solutions can than be evaluated and the patient will be encouraged to select the solution she or he thinks best.

Return to page 233 and try again.

You picked C

Do you have any ideas what you might do about this situation?

This is the correct response. This is an example of a solution-oriented response that helps the speaker to shift from exploration of the problem situation to consideration of possible solutions. This kind of response accomplishes two things: First, it shifts the focus from problem definition to solution orientation. Second, it seeks specific suggestions from the patient. Remember, this type of response is given only after the problem has been fully explored and defined. This might be 15 minutes or 2 hours after the problem was initially introduced.

Proceed to page 237.

Shifting Focus: Exercise 2

Select from the following responses the one that is a solution-oriented response that shifts the focus from exploration of the problem to possible solutions.

> *Tina:*   *My father is changing jobs and wants us to move right away. This is my last year of high school, and I don't want to leave all my friends.*
>
> *Ms. Zachary:*   A. *Where are you moving?*
> B. *Is there anything that could be done about it?*
> C. *Don't worry about it. A person as friendly as you are will make more friends wherever you go.*

If you picked A, turn to page 238.
If you picked B, turn to page 239.
If you picked C, turn to page 240.

You picked A

Where are you moving?

This is not a solution-oriented response because it does not help the patient focus on possible solutions to the problem. This is a questioning response, asking for more information. The nurse is trying to get more information from the patient, possibly so that she can suggest a plausible solution. This is the kind of response that beginning helpers often make. It indicates that the earlier stage of the problem exploration was not given enough attention. It also indicates that the nurse does not respect the patient's ability to solve his or her own problem.

**Return to page 237
and try again.**

You picked B

Is there anything that could be done about it?

Congratulations! You're correct. This is a solution-oriented response that shifts the focus from exploration of the problem to possible solutions. Notice that, although it is phrased as a question, the intent is to help the patient to focus on what might be done to resolve the problem. This kind of response prompts the patient to suggest her own solutions. The solutions she suggests may be ones she thought of on her own or they may have been suggested to her by others. The origin and quality of the solutions is irrelevant as long as the patient assumes some responsibility for the problem and introduces the solutions herself.

Turn to page 241.

You picked C

> *Don't worry about it. A person as friendly as you are will make more friends wherever you go.*

This is not a response that shifts the focus from problem exploration to possible solutions. It is not even a solution-oriented response. This is an example of a response that communicates both a lack of respect for and a lack of understanding of the patient. The phrase "Don't worry about it" discounts the patient's implied feelings of concern. The attempt to reassure the patient by telling her "You will make more friends wherever you go" communicates lack of understanding of Tina's immediate concerns. This patient is concerned about keeping her present friends, not about making new ones.

You were asked to select a solution-oriented response that would help the patient shift the focus from description of the problem to possible solutions; the correct response will help the patient to suggest solutions to the problem she mentioned.

Return to page 237 and try again.

CONSIDERING SPECIFIC SOLUTIONS

Responses that ask the patient to consider a specific solution presented by the nurse should be made only after the patient has been encouraged to suggest all the possible solutions she or he can think of. Only after the patient's repertoire is completely exhausted should the nurse suggest additional alternatives to the patient. The time for the nurse to begin suggesting solutions varies with each situation, but the moment will usually be marked by a statement by the patient such as "I can't think of anything else" or "There aren't any other possibilities."

If, in response to your suggestions, the patient acknowledges your ideas but disputes their value, then most likely you have progressed too rapidly through the stages of problem exploration and definition. Patient responses that can indicate this situation are usually of the form "Yes, but ..." or "Yes, I hear your solution, but it's not a workable one for me."

However, if you've thoroughly worked through the earlier stages of helping, the suggestion of appropriate and relevant alternatives is an easy task. Your suggestions will flow from your understanding of the patient and his or her problem. Relevant and helpful suggestions communicate a deep understanding of the patient and further facilitate the development of the relationship between nurse and patient.

After each suggestion the nurse presents, the patient should be asked to think of any other alternatives. The nurse should encourage the patient to build on the alternatives presented—that is, to suggest new alternatives stimulated by the nurse's ideas. This process of mutual suggestion and problem solving is a very healthy one, but never forget that the major responsibility for problem solving rests with the patient.

This phase of the solution-seeking process is completed when neither the nurse nor the patient can think of any other solutions. When this happens, it's time to move on to phase three of the solution-seeking process—evaluating the alternatives.

Suggesting Specifics: Exercise 1

Consider now the second type of solution-oriented response. Which one of the following responses is an example of a solution-oriented response that suggests specific solutions for the patient to consider?

> *Dave:*　　I'd like to ask the doctor when I'll get to go home, but I'm afraid to ask him. He always acts so busy.
>
> *Ms. Quinn:*　A. Don't be shy. Next time he comes in, ask him.
> 　　　　　　　B. Why are you afraid to ask him?
> 　　　　　　　C. Have you thought about asking your wife to call him at his office and talk to him?

If you picked A, turn to page 243.
If you picked B, turn to page 244.
If you picked C, turn to page 245.

You picked A

Don't be so shy. Next time he comes in, ask him.

    This is not the correct response. This is an example of advice giving—telling the patient what to do. It's not a good solution-oriented response. The patient has indicated that he would like to ask the doctor when he will get to go home but that he's afraid to ask him. "Commanding" Dave to do so probably won't make him any more able to do it. Further, the statement "Don't be so shy" communicates a lack of understanding of and respect for both the patient and his disclosure of fear and apprehension.

    Good solution-oriented responses should be phrased in the form of a suggestion for the speaker's consideration, not as a command. Ms. Quinn should offer solutions for the patient to consider and evaluate. She should not assume that her solution is the best or the only one.

Return to page 242 and try again.

You picked B

Why are you afraid to ask him?

This is a questioning response, asking for more information, rather than a response that helps the speaker to consider a specific solution to the problem. This kind of response is *never* appropriate. "Why" questions seek justification from the patient, assume authority, and serve no facilitative purpose. They make the patient defensive and should always be avoided.

The purpose of solution-oriented responses is not to evaluate the patient's behavior, but rather to help the patient to consider and evaluate possible solutions to the problem presented.

Return to page 242 and try again.

You picked C

Have you thought about asking your wife to call him at his office and talk to him?

This is the correct response. This response suggests a specific solution to be considered by the patient. It suggests only one of many solutions that could have been presented by the nurse. Remember, though, that specific suggestions by the nurse should be made only after the patient has voiced all of his or her own ideas.

Turn to page 246.

Suggesting Specifics: Exercise 2

Consider the following patient's statement and select the nurse's response that is an example of a solution-oriented response that asks the speaker to consider a specific solution.

Harriet Phillips: *My husband went down to check on my hospital bill today. I owe over $3000, and we don't have any insurance.*

Mr. Montez: A. *Have you considered trying to get insurance?*

B. *Have you considered talking to the bookkeeping department about an extended-payment plan?*

C. *Do you have any idea how you will pay the bill?*

If you picked A, turn to page 247.
If you picked B, turn to page 248.
If you picked C, turn to page 249.

You picked A

Have you considered trying to get insurance?

This is not the correct response. It asks Harriet to consider a specific solution, but the solution suggested is not relevant to the problem. Harriet is concerned about paying the hospital the $3000 she now owes. Insurance will not help her with this problem, although it might help her to avoid this problem in the future.

The correct response would suggest a specific solution that is relevant to the problem presented.

Return to page 246 and try again.

You picked B

> *Have you considered talking to the bookkeeping depart-*
> *ment about an extended-payment plan?*

This is the correct response. It suggests a specific solution that is relevant to the problem. This response serves two functions: it provides Harriet with an alternative to consider, and it educates her about a hospital service with which she might not have been familiar.

Turn to page 250.

You picked C

Do you have any idea how you will pay the bill?

This is not the correct response. It is a solution-oriented response, but it's one that would best serve to shift the focus of a discussion from exploration and definition to solution finding; it does not ask the speaker to consider a specific solution. The correct response would suggest a specific solution that is relevant to the problem presented.

Return to page 246 and try again.

EVALUATING THE ALTERNATIVES

The third type of solution-oriented response focuses on the evaluation of alternatives. This type of response asks the patient "What are the advantages and disadvantages of this particular solution?" or "What do you think would happen if you tried this solution?" It helps the patient to evaluate, one by one, all the alternatives presented earlier in the problem-solving process. Discussing each alternative will increase the likelihood that the patient will select the most appropriate solution in this final phase of the problem-solving process.

While the two of you are evaluating solutions, new solutions may occur to you. Because good, workable solutions are often arrived at by modifying previous alternatives, modifications of earlier suggestions also should be encouraged.

The process of evaluating alternatives should begin only after all possible solutions have been suggested. It's important not to overlap the phases of alternative suggestion and alternative evaluation, since the evaluation process will discourage the suggestion of possibly helpful solutions. This third phase of the problem-solving process is completed only after every possible solution has been independently evaluated.

Evaluating Alternatives: Exercise 1

Which of the following responses is an example of a solution-oriented response that helps the speaker to evaluate a solution?

Oliver Klein: *I don't want to go home—not in this wheelchair anyhow. I can't manage without my legs.*

Ms. D'Anuncio: *A. If you don't go home, what else can you do?*

              B. Maybe it would help to explore what would happen if you hired a nurse to stay with you for a while.

              C. How about having your family give you some extra help when you first get home?

If you picked A, turn to page 252.
If you picked B, turn to page 253.
If you picked C, turn to page 254.

You picked A

If you don't go home, what else can you do?

This is not the correct response. This is a solution-oriented response, but it would be better used in shifting the focus of a discussion from problem exploration and definition to consideration of alternatives. It says to the patient "What can you do?"

The correct response should help the patient to consider the options and evaluate the advantages and disadvantages of each.

Return to page 251 and pick the correct response.

You picked B

> *Maybe it would help to explore what would happen if you hired a nurse to stay with you for a while.*

This is the correct response. This is an example of a solution-oriented response that helps the patient to evaluate the consequences of a particular solution. It asks the patient to explore the advantages and disadvantages of this specific solution. The consequences of the solutions presented should always be considered first before moving on to phase four of the problem-solving process.

Turn to page 255.

You picked C

How about having your family give you some extra help when you first get home?

This is a solution-oriented response, but it does not achieve the goal that was specified—helping the patient to evaluate a particular solution. This response asks the speaker to consider a specific solution, not evaluate one.

Return to page 251 and try again.

Evaluating Alternatives: Exercise 2

Read this patient's statement and select the response that is solution oriented and helps the speaker to evaluate a solution.

> *Jackie Tucker:*   *My daughter has to be hospitalized for a long time. I have to decide whether to send her to Good Hope Hospital or to Three Sisters. I don't know what to do.*
>
> *Mr. Venner:*   *A. You should send her to Good Hope. They have a better pediatric department.*
> *B. How do you think things would work out if you chose Three Sisters?*
> *C. Could you visit both Good Hope and Three Sisters and see how you like them?*

If you picked A, turn to page 256.
If you picked B, turn to page 257.
If you picked C, turn to page 258.

You picked A

> **You should send her to Good Hope. They have a better pediatric department.**

This is not a solution-oriented response that helps the patient to evaluate a solution. In addition, notice that the nurse has presented his personal opinion: "You should send her to Good Hope." Statements that tell the patient what should be done are never helpful during any phase of the problem-solving process. This nurse also gave his personal opinion about the quality of care at both the two hospitals: "They [Good Hope] have a better pediatric department [than Three Sisters]." Nursing staff should help the patient explore the possibilities involved but should refrain from providing personal opinions.

Return to page 255 and try again.

You picked B

How do you think things would work if you chose Three Sisters?

This is the correct response. It's an example of a solution-oriented response that helps the speaker to evaluate a specific solution. The nurse's statement, phrased as a question, suggests that the speaker consider the possible consequences of one of the choices. The next step would be to consider the consequences of choosing the other hospital. The consequences of each choice should be considered before the patient makes the decision.

Turn to page 259.

You picked C

Could you visit both Good Hope and Three Sisters and see how you like them?

This is a solution-oriented response, but it is not the type you were asked to pick. This response helps the patient to focus on a specific solution. Notice, though, that the solution is *suggested* by the nurse and not presented as a solution the patient must accept. The suggested solution is a valuable one, since it will eventually help the patient to select a plan of action based on knowledge she obtained herself. However, you were asked to select a solution-oriented response that would help the speaker to consider the consequences of selecting a particular solution.

Return to page 255 and try again.

SELECTING A PLAN OF ACTION

Selecting a plan of action is the final phase of the problem-solving process. The purpose of this phase is to help the patient decide what he or she wants to do about the problem presented. Since it is the last phase of the problem-solving process, it is also intended to provide closure to the entire helping process. Responses in this phase of the process ask the client "What do you want to do about the problem?" Notice that both the decision and responsibility for action rest with the patient; the patient alone will reap the consequences of his or her behavior. The decision to be made in this phase of the process should flow easily from the previous stages if each stage was developed completely. Failure to attend to any of the previous stages of helping will manifest itself in the patient's inability to make a decision in this final stage. And, of course, the patient should not be asked to make a decision until all suggested alternatives have been thoroughly evaluated.

Selecting a Plan: Exercise 1

Read the following statement and select the nurse's response that helps the patient to select a plan of action.

> **Kevin:** *My parents are getting a divorce, and I have to choose which one I want to live with. I don't know what to do.*
>
> **Ms. Evans:** A. *You should stay with your mother. She's going to need someone around the house to help her.*
> B. *How do you think things would work out if you moved in with your father?*
> C. *We've outlined and evaluated just about all your options. What do you think you'd like to do?*

If you picked A, turn to page 261.
If you picked B, turn to page 262.
If you picked C, turn to page 263.

You picked A

> *You should stay with your mother. She's going to need someone around the house to help her.*

This is not a solution-oriented response that helps the speaker to select a plan of action. This response is an example of advice giving. The nurse is selecting a plan of action for the patient, which is contrary to the basis of the entire problem-solving process. The objective of the problem-solving process is for the patient to suggest, evaluate, and select a plan of action, because it is he or she who will have to live with the consequences.

Return to page 260 and try again.

You picked B

How do you think things would work out if you moved in with your father?

This is not a solution-oriented response that helps the patient to select a plan of action. Instead, this response helps the patient to evaluate a particular solution: the nurse's statement suggests that the speaker consider the advantages and disadvantages of living with his father. The correct response would ask the patient to make a decision about whom he wants to live with.

Return to page 260 and try again.

You picked C

> ***We've outlined and evaluated just about all your options.
> What do you think you'd like to do?***

This is the correct response. It asks the patient to select a plan of action. Notice that the responsibility for the selection of a solution and for action rests with the patient. It is the patient who will have to live with the consequences of the decision.

Turn to page 264.

Selecting a Plan: Exercise 2

Read this patient's statement and select the response that helps the patient to select a plan of action.

> **Mrs. Nava:**   *I don't want my husband to see me like this! I'm afraid of losing him. With only one breast, I'm only half a woman.*
>
> **Mr. Schmidt:**   A. *Don't let it get you down. If he really loves you, it won't matter at all.*
>
> B. *Your husband is waiting outside. What do you want to do?*
>
> C. *Do you have any idea what you might do?*

If you picked A, turn to page 265.
If you picked B, turn to page 266.
If you picked C, turn to page 267.

You picked A

Don't let it get you down. If he really loves you, it won't matter at all.

This is not the correct response. This response does not ask the patient to select a plan of action nor does it facilitate the problem-solving process. The response communicates a lack of understanding of and respect for the patient. It says "I don't appreciate your concern and fears."

The correct response would be to ask the patient to select a plan of action. It would say "What do you want to do?"

Return to page 264 and try again.

You picked B

Your husband is waiting outside. What do you want to do?

This is the correct response. It asks the patient to make a decision. It is the conclusion of the problem-solving process.

Turn to page 268.

You picked C

Do you have any idea what you might do?

This is not the correct response. This is a solution-oriented response that asks the patient what she *might* do. It shifts the focus to problem exploration, but it does not ask the patient to make a decision. The correct response would ask the patient to make a decision based on her understanding of the problem, her alternatives, and the consequences of those alternatives.

Return to page 264 and pick the correct response.

SUMMARY

1. Solution-oriented responses should help the patient to engage in the problem-solving process and select a satisfactory solution.
2. There are four types of solution-oriented responses:
   a. Responses that help the patient shift the discussion from exploration of the problem to consideration of solutions.
   b. Responses that help the patient to consider specific solutions suggested by the nurse.
   c. Responses that help the patient to evaluate specific solutions.
   d. Responses that help the patient to select a plan of action.
3. Solution-oriented responses should be phrased as suggestions, such as:
   a. "What do you think you can do about it . . ."
   b. "Have you considered . . ."
   c. "What would happen if . . ."
   d. "What are you going to do about . . ."
4. Solution-oriented responses are not appropriate at the beginning of a conversation with a patient who is presenting a problem. They should be used only after the problem situation has been explored and defined.

9
Interaction Analysis

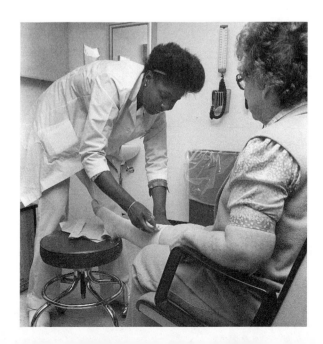

This chapter will give you an opportunity to see in action the principles and techniques you mastered in the previous eight chapters. Five different interactions are presented, each illustrating communication with different types of patients. In situation 1, the problem-solving model is employed to help a patient with a marital problem. Situation 2 illustrates how to talk to children, and situation 3 provides strategies for dealing with the typical angry patient. Situation 4 provides assistance in communicating with relatives, an often neglected area of nursing practice. Finally, situation 5 illustrates strategies for talking to dying patients, especially AIDS patients.

SITUATION 1: THE PROBLEM-SOLVING MODEL

The following is a nurse/patient situation in which the problem-solving model we have outlined is employed. All four stages of the helping process are illustrated. Take note of the beginning and ending of each stage and of how the listener facilitates the transition periods. Notice how reflections, clarifications, and questions are formulated and how the nurse assists the patient to better understand the problem and come to a solution. The nurse/patient interaction is on the left and the analysis of the nurse's responses is on the right.

The Helping Process

Stage 1: Expression/disclosure—begins with statement 1 and closes with statement 17.

Stage 2: Defining the problem—begins with statement 1 and ends with statement 22.

Stage 3: Goal-setting/alternatives—begins with statement 22 and ends with statement 35.

Stage 4: Solution/goal-evaluation—begins with statement 35 and ends with statement 42.

Interaction

1. *P:* Ms. Kogler, may I talk to you a minute?

2. *N:* Sure, Ms. Donaldson. Let me put this chart down and pull up a chair.

3. *P:* Last night when my husband left here, he asked me whether I was doing what the doctor told me.

4. *N:* Your husband asked you whether you were doing what the doctor told you to do?

Analysis

2. *N:* The nurse expresses a positive interest in the patient and her request.

4. *N:* A reflective response, intended to communicate to the patient that the nurse is listening.

Interaction	**Analysis**
5. *P:* Yeah; he was mad because he suspects that I'm not cooperating.	
6. *N:* Your husband was mad because he thinks that you aren't cooperating with your doctor.	6. *N:* A reflection of the patient's reference to her husband's feelings.
7. *P:* Was he! He started yelling at me the minute he walked in the door. I just couldn't stand it.	
8. *N:* You don't like it when your husband yells at you.	8. *N:* Reflection of the patient's feelings to promote further disclosure of these feelings.
9. *P:* No, I don't. He thinks I'm no good. He just doesn't understand me.	
10. *N:* Your husband doesn't understand you?	10. *N:* Reflection of the content of the patient's message. Notice how the nurse chose to reflect the patient's general concern at the lack of her husband's understanding. This prompts the patient to talk more about her relationship with her husband (statement 11). Reflection of the husband's opinion of his wife would have resulted in a discussion of the negative

Interaction	**Analysis**
	interactions, which seems less crucial at this time.
11. *P:* No, he doesn't. I'd like him to be proud of me, but instead he's ashamed of me.	
12. N: It hurts that your husband's ashamed of you.	12. *N:* Clarification of patient's response. The nurse focuses on the patient's implied feeling of hurt and prompts further disclosure on the part of the patient. A reflection such as "You'd like your husband to be proud of you" would also have been helpful but probably would not have prompted the same depth of response (statement 13).
13. *P:* It does. I want him to love me so much [crying], but nothing I ever do seems good enough! I try so hard to please him.	
14. *N:* You really want your husband's love, but nothing you do seems to please him.	14. *N:* A reflection of both the patient's desire for her husband's love and her efforts to please him. The patient can choose to respond to either of these elements.

Interaction	**Analysis**
15. P: Nothing. I try to do things to make him happy, but nothing seems to work. One day I cooked a special dish he loves that his mother always cooked for him—something he's talked about and wanted for a long time—but all he did was scream at me for wasting time. He said it didn't taste right anyway.	15. N: The patient chooses to elaborate on her attempts at pleasing her husband, the less threatening of the two topics.
16. N: Even when you do things you think will please him, he's not satisfied.	16. N: A reflection of the patient's general concern. Notice that the nurse does not discuss the specific example mentioned by the patient.
17. P: That's right. I just don't know what to do.	
18. N: You need help with two problems right now. You're concerned that your husband thinks you're not cooperating with your medical treatment, and, at a deeper level, you're worried that your husband doesn't love you because nothing you do seems to please him. Which do you want to talk about now?	18. N: A summarization by the nurse. It says to the patient "This is where we are; where do you want to go from here?" Notice how the choice of direction is left up to the patient.

Interaction	**Analysis**
19. *P:* I'm really concerned about my relationship with my husband and how that might be improved. But I don't think we can do anything about that right now. Anyway, at this moment I'm really scared about what my husband will say when he finds out that I lied to him and haven't really been doing what the doctor says I should.	
20. *N:* You're afraid that your husband will find out that you weren't honest with him and that he'll be upset with you.	20. *N:* Reflection of what the patient describes as her present concern. Notice that this is a shift from initial reflection of the patient's feelings.
21. *P:* Yes, I am. I think he might ask you or one of the other nurses. Then what will I do? He'll know that I lied.	
22. *N:* The problem that seems to be concerning you is the aftereffects of your dishonesty. Let's think of some way you could deal with those consequences.	22. *N:* The nurse first reflects the problem and then shifts the focus to the listing of possible solutions.
23. *P:* Well, maybe my husband will avoid the whole problem then. He's never find out	

Interaction	Analysis
that I lied. And I'll start doing what I'm supposed to do.	
24. *N:* He would never find out unless one of us told him.	24. *N:* A poor response by the nurse. It is threatening to the patient because it implies "I'm going to tell your husband that you lied." It puts distance between nurse and patient, and causes the patient to wonder "Why did I trust this person with my problems?" A better response would have been "Maybe your husband will never call me, and then this whole incident will blow over."
25. *P:* You wouldn't do that would you? You wouldn't call him up and tell him?	25. *N:* The nurse's response has prompted defensiveness on the part of the patient. The patient immediately feels inferior to the nurse and asks her not to disclose her secret.
26. *N:* No, I wouldn't, not unless you and I decided that it was the best solution.	26. *N:* The nurse notices the patient's defensive reaction. She tries to reassure the patient that she will not betray her trust. She is able to do this only because their relationship has been firmly established.

Interaction

Analysis

27. *P:* Well it's not. He'd be madder than ever finding it out from you.

28. *N:* How else might we attack this problem?

28. *N:* A question that attempts to solicit patient suggestions. Notice that the nurse has not suggested solutions.

29. *P:* Well, I could tell him the truth—that I just haven't had the energy to do those exercises and that they hurt too much. But he doesn't like weak people.

30. *N:* Can you think of any other solutions?

30. *N:* Another attempt to prompt the patient for solutions.

31. *P:* If he asks you about me, you could lie. You could tell him that I really have been cooperating.

32. *N:* Can you think of any other possibilities?

32. *N:* Another prompt.

33. *P:* Well, I guess you could tell him the truth if he asks you.

34. *N:* Let's see; we've listed five possibilities. You could call your husband and tell him the truth, or I could call him up and try to

34. *N:* A summarization of the solution presented combined with a final attempt to solicit any further ideas.

Interaction

Analysis

explain the situation
to him. Or, we can
hope that he doesn't
ask me and just let the
whole situation blow
over. If he does ask
me, I can either tell
the truth or lie. Can
you think of any other
possibilities?

35. *P:* No, not really.

36. *N:* Then which of these
five solutions you've
suggested do you think
is best?

36. *N:* A questions that seeks
the patient's evalua-
tion of the solutions
presented. Notice that
the nurse refrains from
evaluating the solu-
tions. However, the
nurse could have pro-
vided information
about her willingness
or unwillingness to lie
for the patient or to
contact the patient's
husband.

37. *P:* I don't know. I know I
don't think it's fair of
me to ask you to lie. I
really wouldn't want
you to do that.

38. *N:* Well, how do you feel
about the other
possibilities?

38. *N:* Another question that
asks the patient to
evaluate the solutions
presented.

39. *P:* I guess I don't want to
count on his not
asking about it. And I
don't want him not to
know; I'd always be

Interaction	**Analysis**
afraid that he would eventually find out somehow. Anyway, that's a copout, trying to keep him from knowing.	
40. *N:* You'd like your husband to know the truth, but you're still not sure how you want him to find out. Either one of us could tell him.	40. *N:* A clarification of the patient's present position. It presents the patient with the final choice. By clarifying the patient's position, the nurse hastens the helping process.
41. *P:* It would be easier to have you tell him, but I think it would be best if it came from me. I want to try to start having a more honest relationship with my husband. Anyway, I want to tell him how important he is to me.	
42. *N:* I think you've made a wise decision. Be sure to let me know how everything comes out. If you run into a problem, we can work on it together.	42. *N:* Another critical response. Here the nurse closes the discussion by communicating two important things to the patient. She communicates her support and she invites her to talk again, opening the door for further communication.
43. *P:* I will. Thank you so much.	

SITUATION 2: CHILDREN AS PATIENTS

Communicating with children poses a unique challenge to the medical community. Children are psychologically and intellectually different from their adult counterparts. Children are more dependent, less verbal, more open, less intellectual, more literal, and more emotional than adults. Nurses who work with children must keep these differences in mind when communicating with children. Here are a few points to consider:

• Children think of themselves as invincible and they are easily upset when their bodies don't work right. When anything goes wrong, even something as simple as a cavity or pimple, it unnerves them because it shatters the premise that they are invincible. They view themselves as young and strong; they are not supposed to get sick. When talking with children about their illness, remember how frightened they are and proceed slowly. Emphasize the duration of the disease and their recovery, when realistic.

• Children have a short attention span. The younger the child, the shorter the attention span. Keep explanations short and to the point to help children understand them. In conjunction with their short attention span, children hate to be confined. Confinement is equated with lack of stimulation and boredom. Consequently, long hospital stays are difficult for children and often lead to depression.

• Children have a limited ability to understand abstract concepts. They are concrete rather than abstract in their thinking. Time is a particularly difficult concept for young children to understand. Consequently, when they are told, "This will burn for 30 seconds," or "You should feel better in three days," that is often not much reassurance. When referencing time, help children understand the duration in question.

• Children have a limited vocabulary. They often have difficulty understanding concepts because they don't understand the words used to explain them. Explain concepts to children in clear and simple terms. Use short sentences and frequently check if you are being understood.

• Children are visually rather than verbally oriented. If you approach a child with a hypodermic needle and say, "It won't hurt," the child will probably start to scream. To capitalize on children's beliefs in what they see rather than what they hear, use props when explaining procedures to children. Demonstrate on your self or on a doll to help reduce anxiety.

• Children have limited exposure to the medical community. Routine exams can frighten them because they are unfamiliar. Ask children if they have had the procedure in question before. If not, explain it very carefully. If children do have significant exposure to a hospital, it is generally vicarious. For example, grandma went to the hospital and she died there, or grandpa went to the hospital and he had an operation. When admitted to a hospital, children draw on these experiences and naturally wonder, "Am I going to have an operation?" or "Am I going to die?" When working with children, find out if they have visited any close relatives in the hospital. Such information may help you better understand the child's hidden fears.

Here are some guidelines to use when talking to children:

Talk at a level children can understand. Children need and want information. The four questions most commonly asked by children are: (1) What's wrong with me? (2) How did I get it? (3) How long will it last? and (4) Will it hurt? In medical terms, they want to know the nature of the disease, how it was contracted, its duration, and its symptoms. When faced with any new procedure, children want to know, "What are you going to do?" and "Will it hurt?" Even routine procedures like a blood pressure test or a TB test can scare children on the first exposure. Be sensitive to their age. Provide answers in clear and simple language. Don't distort information to simplify it.

Tell the truth. Nurses who would never think of lying to adult patients will lie to children to spare them from the truth. Nurses most frequently lie when they are asked, "Will it hurt?" When children realize that it *does* hurt, they feel a double injustice—it hurt and you lied to them. Once you lie to a child, it's almost impossible to regain his or her trust. The child who suffers unexpected pain at your expense will never forgive you. Next time you approach that same child with a simple procedure, he or she won't believe it's painless and may be difficult to handle.

Don't make empty promises. Promises and children seem to go together. Parents, teachers, and nurses make promises to children to get them to behave. Children, quick to catch on to this relationship, readily extract promises from adults. Don't make a promise that you aren't 100% certain you can keep. If you do make a promise to a child, remember that he or she will take that promise literally. Don't promise ice cream at "7 o'clock" or to "read a story this afternoon"—children aren't tolerant if an emergency arises. It would be better to promise, "I'll read you a story this afternoon if I have time" or "I'll bring you ice cream between 7:00 and 8:00."

Respect the child's feelings. Children are generally open about expressing their feelings. It's not uncommon to hear a child say, "I'm scared," or to start crying. Don't belittle the child's feelings with statements like, "You're a big boy. Act brave," or "Cheer up. There's nothing to cry about." Instead, acknowledge the child's fears or concerns.

Ask questions. The increased use of questions, most notably open-ended questions, is the easiest way to facilitate communication with children. Direct questions—questions that focus on retrieving specific information—can also be helpful. Closed questions—questions that require only a yes or no answer—are less helpful. They encourage brief responses and give the child the impression that you are interrogating him or her.

Here is a dialogue between a nurse and an eight-year-old child. The child is hospitalized with a knee injury and will have surgery in the morning. It's bedtime and the child wants his mother. The nurse, walking by the child's room, sees him crying. She sits on the side of the bed and makes contact.

Pay careful attention to how the nurse helps the child cope with his fears by helping him express them, and then provides the child with acknowledgment and reassurance. Also notice the high frequency of questions.

Interaction	**Analysis**
N: Jimmy, what's wrong?	*N:* An open invitation to talk.
P: (Sobbing) Nothing.	
N: Come on, tell me what's upsetting you.	*N:* A second inquiry into the problem.
P: I want my mommy.	
N: You wish your mother was here. Where is your mother? I saw her here a few minutes ago.	*N:* The nurse reflects the patient's statement and then follows the reflection with a question.
P: She went home. She had to go home to take care of my little brother and sister. I wish she was here with me.	
N: Your mother would like to be here with you but she had to go home and take care of your little brother and sister. They're too young to take care of themselves.	*N:* Nurse elaborates on the patient's explanation of why his mother isn't there.
P: I guess. She could have gotten someone else to take care of them. I need her here with me. I'm scared.	
N: You wish your mother was here to take care of you because you're scared. What are you scared of?	*N:* The nurse acknowledges the patient's fear, then seeks a clarification of it.
P: The operation.	

Interaction

N: You're scared of the operation you're going to have. What scares you?

P: (Child bursts into tears) They're going to cut open my leg tomorrow morning. It's going to hurt. What if I won't be able to walk again?

N: Jimmy, you're afraid it's going to hurt. It won't hurt. You won't even feel it. You'll be sound asleep.

P: What if I wake up?

N: You're afraid you'll wake up in the middle of the operation. Tomorrow, when you go down to the operating room, the doctor will give you some medicine to put you to sleep. You'll sleep much deeper than you do at night. Even the operation won't wake you up.

P: Are you sure ?

N: I'm sure. Is there anything else that scares you about the operation?

P: What if I can't walk? They're cutting my leg

Analysis

N: The nurse acknowledges the child's fear and then asks for further clarification of it.

N: The nurse now understands the patient's fears and she can begin to reassure him.

N: The nurse acknowledges the patient's fear and then continues to reassure him.

N: The nurse prompts the patient to disclose any other fears so that she can reassure him.

Interaction	**Analysis**
open, aren't they? What if they mess it up?	
N: You're worried that you won't be able to walk after the operation. Dr. Hershberger is only going to make a small cut near your knee. She has done this operation many times before. I don't think there will be a problem.	*N:* The nurse paraphrases the patient's fear and then reassures him.
P: Have you ever had surgery?	
N: I remember I had my tonsils out when I was a little younger than you. I was scared, too, but I was surprised at how easy it was once it was over.	*N:* The nurse relates a story to the patient. The key elements of the story are: she was scared; and even though she was younger, she survived; and it wasn't bad.
P: It won't be bad?	
N: No, it won't be bad. After surgery, you'll be good as new—better, in fact. Now, do you feel better?	*N:* The nurse reassures the patient.
P: Yeah. Can I call my mom?	
N: Sure.	
P: I want to tell her good night.	

SITUATION 3: ANGRY PATIENTS

Dealing with an angry patient is a challenge to any nurse. The natural reaction to anger, or any perceived threat, is to get away from the person who is angry or to fight back. The intensity of this reaction is related to the degree of threat perceived. In a professional role, neither of these responses is satisfactory. Instead, the nurse must dissipate the anger and resolve the conflict.

Here are some tips for communicating with angry patients. When confronted with an angry patient, remember the four Ds: Dissipate, Dispel, Deal, and Direct.

Dissipate the anger first.   The first step in dealing with an angry patient is to diffuse the anger. When a person is angry, emotion rules. You cannot solve the patient's problem or be helpful in any other way until the patient's anger is diffused and the intellect regains control. Anger makes people irrational.

It's not hard to help someone else let go of their anger if you stay calm and remember the following five rules:

1. Acknowledge the patient's right to be angry. All people have a right to be angry, just as they have a right to be happy, sad, or scared. Acknowledge a person's right to be angry, even if you don't agree with his or her reasons for being angry.
2. Show the patient you understand why he or she is angry. Even if you don't agree with the patient's reasons for being angry, it's important that you acknowledge them. Repeat the patient's reasons back to him or her.
3. Don't argue with the patient. Arguing only fuels anger. The more you disagree with angry patients, the more they explain themselves and the more entrenched they become that their position is correct. Don't point out where their information is wrong or where they are illogical. Just listen. Remember, if you argue with a patient, even if you win, you lose.
4. Don't get defensive. Getting defensive is a natural reaction to anger, just like it's a natural reaction to put up your hand if someone throws a punch or to wink when something is headed toward your eye. Counteracting any of these natural tendencies takes concentrated effort. Work at not letting yourself get defensive.
5. Be careful not to defend your coworkers. Frequently patients complain to the nurse about a fellow nurse, their doctor, or other hospital professionals. Do not react by defending your co-

workers; instead, acknowledge the patient's anger and his or her reasons for getting angry.

Dispel misconceptions.   Is the patient's anger based on any misconceptions? Did the patient misunderstand the facts, methods, or goals of treatment? A patient may get angry because he thinks his medication should have been administered every three hours when it was prescribed for every four. Or a patient may have thought the doctor ordered an X-ray, and she's mad at you for not taking her down to X-ray when in reality an X-ray was never ordered. Once misconceptions are clarified, the problem is resolved.

Remember, don't try to clarify misconceptions until the patient's anger is dissipated. If you try to clarify a misconception too soon, the patient's defensiveness and pride will force him or her to argue with you.

Deal with complaints that are under your control.   If the patient's anger is not based on a misconception, he or she may have a legitimate complaint. Is the complaint about something under your control? If it is, deal with it. Don't make empty promises, however acknowledge the legitimacy of the patient's complaint and explain what you're willing to do to rectify the situation. For example, if the patient is angry about a noisy roommate who prevents him or her from getting sleep, see if there is an empty bed, and ask your supervisor if you can transfer the patient.

Direct the patient when dealing with conflicts outside of your range of control.   Often the patient will complain about situations that are outside of your control, such as the wrong meal, waiting two hours for an X-ray, or a son who doesn't visit. In these cases, direct the patient to take action, if possible. Some patients are too sick to act directly, but most can make a call to the kitchen, write a note to the head of X-ray, or call an absent son. Encouraging a patient to take action for himself or herself communicates that you care, and it fosters independence.

The following dialogue is between a nurse and an angry patient. The patient is a 44-year-old woman who has been hospitalized for a compressed disk. She will be in traction for one week in effort to avoid surgery. Because she is immobile and experiencing some pain, she is quick to anger. In this dialogue, the patient confronts the nurse directly after calling her several times on her call button. The nurse resists getting defensive or angry at the patient, even though the patient attacks her directly.

Interaction	Analysis
N: Hi. Did you need something?	*N:* The nurse inquires why the patient called.
P: Do I need something? Yeah, I need something. I need to go to the bathroom. You're lucky I have a strong bladder or you'd have to change the sheets, too.	*P:* The patient, obviously angry, responds sarcastically.
N: You're angry because I didn't come right away.	*N:* The nurse reflects the patient's anger.
P: Right away? I called you four times. Do you think I like having to depend on you to go to the bathroom or to get a drink of water?	
N: You'd rather do things by yourself, but you can't.	*N:* The nurse reflects the patient's frustration.
P: You know I can't— that's why I don't understand why you don't come sooner. You just sit out there and talk with your friends when you know I need help. I can't believe nurses are so insensitive. Why did you pick nursing, anyway, if you didn't want to help people?	

Interaction	Analysis
N: You're angry at me because you think I spend time talking to my friends rather than doing my job.	*N:* In an effort to dissipate the patient's anger, the nurse avoids getting angry. Instead, she reflects the content of the patient's statement, using the expression, "you think."
P: Well, isn't your job to help patients? Something's wrong if I have to call four times to get some attention around here. What if I didn't have to go to the bathroom? What if I was choking or couldn't breathe? What then?	
N: You think you don't get enough attention. You would like me to respond quicker when you call.	*N:* The nurse avoids responding to the personal attacks. Instead, she responds to the patient's need for more attention.
P: Yes, I would.	*P:* The patient's anger is dissipating.
N: I'll try to respond quicker. I was just down the hall trying to help a patient who was in a lot of pain. I'm sorry I kept you waiting.	*N:* This response has three key components. First, the nurse hears the patient's request and makes a commitment to change. Second, she dispels the misconception

Interaction	Analysis
	that she was sitting and talking to her friends. Third, she took responsibility for her behavior by apologizing.
P: That's OK. It's just that when no one comes when I call, I feel no one cares.	
N: You feel forgotten when no one comes when you call.	*N:* The nurse could have ended the conversation here, by responding with, "I'm glad you feel better now," or "I'm glad we got this resolved." Instead, she decided to pursue the conversation.
P: I feel like I'm in a cave back here. I'm an active person. I'm not used to lying on my back all day, doing nothing.	
N: You're bored here alone in the hospital all day.	*N:* The nurse clarifies the patient's statement and adds the word *alone* since she knows the woman has not had many visitors.
P: It's hard. I'm supposed to be resting, but I'm not tired.	

Interaction	Analysis
N: Would you like to have a room closer to the nurses' station? There's a lot more action up there. At least there would be something to see.	*N:* The nurse suggests a solution to help decrease the patient's loneliness.
P: I'd like that. It's boring back here. I feel like I'm in a cave.	
N: I'll go see if there are any free rooms, or if there is another patient who would like to move back here where it's quieter. I'll let you know.	*N:* The nurse checks immediately. Even if a switch is not possible, the patient knows the nurse cares.
P: Thanks for checking.	

SITUATION 4: COMMUNICATING WITH RELATIVES

A visit to any doctor's waiting room or to a hospital floor will find relatives trying to comfort, entertain, or just offer their presence as reassurance to sick relatives. These relatives range from young children visiting their sick mother, adult children visiting an elderly parent, a wife visiting her dying husband, a mother nurturing her sick child, to sisters, brothers, aunts, and uncles. Other visitors, not true relatives, may also have a close relationship with the patient that warrants respect: a gay man visiting his lover who has AIDS, a live-in boyfriend, a long-time roommate, or a neighbor of 20 years. All of these "relatives" want information and reassurance. Talking to relatives is a central component in the care of a patient.

When treating a minor, it is general practice to discuss the treatment with the child's parent or guardian, in addition to the child. In certain situations, it is also wise to discuss the treatment plan with the patient's relatives. Working in partnership with the patient's family can increase compliance, improve communication, and reduce the anxiety of the patient and the relatives.

Relatives frequently complain that they are ignored by the nursing staff when visiting the patient in the hospital. Nurses, often overwhelmed and overworked, are seldom more than polite to relatives, whom they view as demanding additional time and attention. Relatives ask questions, demand services for the patient, get in the way when the patient is being treated, and are quick to question the treatment plan. In spite of these liabilities, talking to the patient's relatives can be in everyone's best interest. If managed correctly, relatives can be a tremendous resource to the nursing staff and provide assistance in a variety of areas to the patient.

Relatives are the liaison between the patient, the medical staff, and the rest of the family. When a patient is seriously ill, a close relative generally becomes responsible for interfacing between the patient and the rest of the family. All calls from family and friends are usually routed to that relative. A well-informed relative who has confidence in the medical team can reassure the rest of the family that the loved one is well cared for. This vote of confidence from a valued family member can save the nursing staff both time and aggravation.

When a patient is seriously ill, is a minor, or is elderly, then relatives often make decisions regarding the treatment of the patient. Even fully competent adult patients generally discuss their case with friends and relatives and seek their advice and consultation. Informed relatives can be more helpful in the decision-making process than relatives who are basing their opinions on suppositions and thirdhand reports.

Relatives are often responsible for the care of the patient after he or she leaves the hospital. Current insurance regulations and the cost of hospitalization require that patients leave the hospital sooner than ever. When the patient leaves the hospital, it is often a relative who cares for the patient until the individual is well enough to care for himself or herself. A well-informed relative who understands the treatment plan and feels like a partner in the treatment of the patient can take better care of a loved one than a relative who is expected to administer medications or follow directions blindly.

Anxiety not only makes a patient difficult to care for but it can be counterproductive to recovery. A calm relative can ease the concerns of an anxious patient, whereas an anxious relative can raise the anxiety level of a patient. Relatives who stay in the patient's room and make comments like, "I don't know why they don't try ..." or "Where is your doctor?" can raise the anxiety level of patients.

Relatives can ease the burden on the nursing staff. By providing the patient with companionship and helping the patient with routine needs, an informed relative can save a busy nursing staff a tremendous amount of time, as well as boost the patient's morale.

Although talking with relatives can be a time-consuming proposition for nurses, the benefits far outweigh the investment. When talking with relatives, keep in mind these five simple guidelines.

Listen to relatives. Be sensitive to the emotional needs of the patient's family. Fear, concern, depression, anger, and guilt are all feelings commonly experienced when a loved one is ill. Overwhelmed by these emotions, loved ones often hide them so as not to upset the patient. Trying to hide their feelings from the patient and being physically exhausted from taking care of the patient places a tremendous emotional strain on relatives. Consequently, their feelings are often vented inappropriately at the medical staff. Instead of getting defensive, treat relatives with respect. Hear what the relatives have to say before the situation reaches a crisis level. Use the same listening techniques and strategies you use with your patients.

Know the policy regarding talking to relatives.   Patients have a right to privacy. Just because a relative drives the patient to the office or visits a patient in the hospital does not give that relative automatic access to privileged information about the patient. A nurse is constantly forced to make decisions regarding with whom to discuss the patient's case. The nurse's decision should be influenced by organizational policy as well as by the age of the patient and the severity of the patient's illness. Parents have access to information about minors, and adult children generally are given information regarding their infirmed parents. Generally, relatives are given more information about seriously ill patients than less ill ones.

Ask the patient for permission to discuss his or her health with relatives or friends.   Often friends and relatives ask the nurse for information when the patient is too sick, too drugged, too young, or for some other reason incapable of explaining current problems. If none of these situations is the case, the relative or friend may be asking for information because the patient is intentionally withholding such information. Under these circumstances, before you reveal confidential information, ask the patient's permission to talk to a relative or friend. If the patient says no, respect this request.

Answer questions openly and honestly.   Once you establish that you are not violating the patient's privacy, answer questions openly and honestly. Relatives' concerns are genuine and their need for information is real. Information reduces their anxiety and helps them cope with the illness of a loved one. The more information a relative has, the greater assistance he or she can provide in the care of the patient.

Advise relatives to discuss the patient's case with his or her doctor.   When the patient's relatives ask for a justification of the treatment plan or ask for an evaluation of the quality of the patient's care, advise them to discuss the case with the patient's doctor. Some doctors are willing to discuss the patient's case at the hospital. Others are only willing to talk briefly at the hospital and prefer long conversations to occur in the office. If relatives complain that a doctor is evasive at the hospital, advise them to schedule an office consultation.

Here is another situation that uses the problem-solving model. This dialogue is between a member of the patient's family and a nurse. The patient, a 60-year-old female, had a radical mastectomy two years ago. Testing revealed that the cancer has spread to her lungs, bone, and brain. She is currently hospitalized for additional treatment.

See if you can identify the four stages of the helping process.

Stage 1: Expression/Disclosure
Stage 2: Defining the Problem
Stage 3: Goal Setting
Stage 4: Solution/Goal Evaluation

Interaction

R: Nurse, can I talk to you for a minute? I need some advice.

N: Sure. Let's go sit in the lounge where we can talk privately.

R: So much is happening with my mother. Everything's happening so fast. I don't know what to do. My mom's just finished chemotherapy and now her doctor has ordered radiation. She gets respiratory treatments and

Analysis

N: The nurse responds positively to a relative's request. By suggesting they go to the lounge, the nurse is implying that she is willing to take the time to listen.

Interaction	Analysis
physical therapy. She's taking so many drugs. I can't keep track of what's what. I wouldn't mind if she was getting better, but she just seems to be getting worse. I don't know if this is the right treatment plan for her.	
N: You're really worried about your mom. She seems to be getting worse even though she's receiving a variety of treatments and medication.	*N:* A clarification of the relative's concerns.
R: Of course I'm worried. Yesterday my mother had blood in her urine. Today she's crying that she's in agony. Everyday it's something. Will it ever end?	
N: Everyday there's another crisis. Today you had to watch your mother suffer.	*N:* A reflection of the relative's concern.
R: When I hear her scream or cry, it rips my insides out. She begs me to help. "Alberta, do something," she cries. "I can't take much more! My back hurts so badly." How would you like to hear your mother cry? It would drive you crazy too. I want to help, but I don't know what to do. It's not the middle ages. The doctor should be able to give her	

Interaction	**Analysis**
something to ease her pain.	
N: You'd like to help your mom feel less pain, but you don't know how or what to do. You spend time with her and show her you care, but you want to do more than that.	*N:* A clarification that emphasizes the reasons for the relative's concerns.
R: I want to make sure she's getting the best care possible. She's too drugged to know what's going on. I feel it's up to me to make decisions, but I don't have enough information to make the right ones.	
N: You feel like you have to manage your mother's treatment.	*N:* A reflection of the relative's feelings of responsibility.
R: Of course I do, and she's too sick and too drugged to know what's best for her. She'll agree to anything the doctor says. My parents are divorced, so my mom doesn't want my father to have any input into what happens to her. I'm the oldest, so everyone looks to me to make decisions.	
N: You feel that since you are the oldest child, it's up to you to make sure your mother gets the best care possible.	*N:* Another reflection of the daughter's belief that it is up to her to manage her mother's treatment plan.

Interaction

Analysis

R: It *is* up to me. I try my
   best, but it's so frustra-
   ting. I want to talk to her
   doctor, but he's so hard to
   reach. He flies in here at 7
   a.m. and is gone by 7:10.
   I don't get here until 8:30
   because I have to get my
   kids breakfast and off to
   school first. By the time I
   get here, he's finished his
   rounds and has left.
   Maybe he talks things
   over with my mom. I don't
   know. If he does, she's too
   drugged to remember.
   Every time I tried to call
   him at his office he's
   either out of the office or
   with a patient. He doesn't
   return my calls when I'm
   still at the number I leave
   with his receptionist.We're
   paying him thousands of
   dollars. You'd think that
   he could at least tell me
   what's going on.

N: You're frustrated because
   you never get a chance to
   talk to your mother's
   doctor.

N: A reflection that clarifies
   the central problem and
   the source of the
   daughter's frustration.

R: Even when I do get to talk
   to him, he doesn't say
   anything. I hired a baby-
   sitter one morning so I
   could be here when he got
   here. He strolled into my

Interaction	**Analysis**
mother's room at 7:00, right on schedule, and asked her how she felt. She looked at him and answered, "Good, good, good." The woman's dying and complains she is in constant pain, yet when he asks her how she feels, she smiles and says, "Good, good, good." He looked at her chart for a brief minute, jotted something in it, and started to leave. I stood so I could talk to him on his way out. I said how worried I was about my mom. He was obviously annoyed by the intrusion. I was interrupting his sacred schedule. He listened to my comments, pretending interest, and told me he was doing everything he could. The conversation lasted less than two minutes. I was getting nowhere, learning nothing. I thought, why bother?	
N: Even when you do get a chance to talk to your mother's doctor, you don't feel satisfied with the information you are getting.	*N:* A reflection that further defines the problem.
R: He doesn't tell me what I need to know. He doesn't explain to me what he's doing or why he's doing it. I guess he just expects me	

Interaction

Analysis

to trust him. But I don't.
My mother's just another
patient to him, but she's
my mother—the only
mother I've got. Why can't
he be more open with me?
Why doesn't he share
what's going on with me?

N: You'd feel better if you
knew more about your
mother's treatment. You'd
like to talk to your
mother's doctor in detail
about her case, but he
doesn't seem willing to do
so. You've tried calling his
office or waiting for him
when he sees your
mother, but neither of
those strategies seemed to
have worked. Do you have
any other ideas?

N: A reflection that restates
the central problem, com-
bined with a prompt for
potential solutions. This
response moves the coun-
seling process from stage
2 to stage 3 of the helping
process.

R: I guess I could switch
doctors. He isn't the only
doctor that treats cancer
patients at this hospital.

N: You've thought about
switching doctors. Do you
have any other ideas?

N: This response para-
phrases one potential
solution offered by the
relative, as well as
prompts her for further
ideas.

R: Well, I could get my sister
and brother to come with
me to the hospital one
morning so that the three

Interaction	**Analysis**
of us could confront him. I think he would be less likely to run out so fast if we were all here.	
N: You, your brother, and your sister could all meet your mother's doctor here one morning to find out about your mother's treatment. Or you could call his office and schedule a consultation with him. He would have more time to talk during a scheduled appointment.	N: This response paraphrases the relative's suggestion. In addition, the nurse subtly suggests that the meeting takes place at the doctor's office rather than at the hospital.
R: Well, if we talked to him at his office, my mother wouldn't be able to hear the conversation.	
N: You now have three possibilities: change doctors, talk to the doctors here, or make an appointment at his office. Do you have any other ideas?	N: This response summarizes all of the relative's suggestions made thus far and prompts for further ideas.
R: I guess I could write a letter to the hospital administrator or to the state medical board. But by the time they did anything, if they did anything, it would be too late for my mother.	
N: You're so frustrated with your mother's doctor that you'd like to complain to anyone who would listen, but you don't think it will	N: This response reflects a new solution and prompts for further suggestions.

Interaction	**Analysis**
do much good. Do you have any other ideas that might help your mother and help you feel better?	
R: The only other thing I've thought about is getting a second opinion. I could make a copy of my mother's chart and pay another oncologist to review it and give an opinion. If the new doctor thought this doctor was doing a good job, I'd feel better.	
N: You would be reassured by having a second opinion that agreed with the current treatment. You'd get the second opinion by asking another oncologist to review your mother's chart at his office. Or you could ask that the oncologist visit her here. A second opinion is a positive suggestion that would make you feel better about her treatment. Do you have any other ideas?	*N:* This response clarifies the relative's suggestion. It adds the idea of having another doctor actually examine the patient rather than just review the chart.
R: Not really.	
N: You've made a lot of positive suggestions. Let's see if I remember them all. You've suggested changing doctors; talking to your mother's doctor	*N:* This response bridges stages 3 and 4 of the helping process. It summarizes all the potential solutions suggested by the relative and asks

Interaction

    here or at his office,
perhaps with your brother
and sister; writing letters
of complaint; and arrang-
ing for a second opinion
by another oncologist. I
think you're so frustrated
that you will want to take
some action, but it's im-
portant to consider each
of your options wisely.
Let's consider them one at
a time. What are the
advantages of switching
doctors?

R: I'd like to switch doctors
because I'm so frustrated
with this guy. But I don't
know if switching doctors
will do any good. My
mother's used to him and
she's been going to him
for almost three years. A
change would probably
upset her. Plus it would
take another doctor time
to become familiar with
her case. What the doctor
is doing may be the right
thing. It's just that I don't
know what his treatment
plan is until after the fact.
He doesn't keep me in-
formed. He tells my
mother very little and she
isn't able to pass it on to
me. Yet, another doctor
may do the same thing.

Analysis

    her to evaluate each re-
sponse independently.

Interaction	**Analysis**
N: You've thought about changing doctors, but you need more information first. A change would be likely to upset her, so you don't want to switch unless you're sure that the new doctor would be more open for communication with you and would be giving her the best treatment.	*N:* This response reflects the relative's evaluation of the effect of switching doctors.
R: I guess I should wait a little longer until I make a decision about switching. At least I want to talk to her doctor about it first.	
N: Your second and third suggestions involved talking to her doctor. You just said you wanted to talk to him before making any decision to switch. Now you just have to decide where to talk, here or at his office.	*N:* This response asks the relative to evaluate whether to talk to the doctor at the hospital or at his office.
R: I've tried talking to him here at the hospital and all I've been is frustrated. Maybe he's more personable and less abrupt at his office. I suppose I'm going to have to pay for a consultation, but it's probably worth it in the long run.	
N: You've decided to talk to her doctor at his office. If you call his receptionist	*N:* This response suggests a strategy for implementing a potential solution.

Interaction	Analysis
and ask her to schedule an appointment that fits your schedule and his, you should have better luck in getting information.	
R: I'll call his office today since I'd really like to get an appointment as soon as possible.	
N: You also suggested writing letters to complain. Are you still considering doing that?	N: Although inappropriately phrased, because it contains a hidden value judgment, this response asks the relative to determine the pros and cons of writing the letters of complaint.
R: I'd like to complain to let someone know that I don't think her doctor is forthcoming with necessary information for the family. But I don't think I'll complain right now. He might find out and it might cause him to be even more distant, or to treat me worse.	
N: You're afraid complaining will only make the situation worse.	N: This response reflects the relative's concerns.
R: Well, I'm sure he wouldn't like me any better if I complained. Anyway, I don't have the time or the energy to complain to anyone right now.	

Interaction

N: You'd like to complain to someone about him, but lack of time and energy holds you back.

R: I might complain after this is all over. If I'm this dissatisfied, I should switch doctors rather than complain. I'll wait until after I talk to him and then decide.

N: You're going to decide what to do after you meet with your mother's doctor.

R: I guess a lot is resting on that meeting.

N: Your last idea was to get a second opinion. What are your reasons for pursuing that?

R: I need the peace of mind that the treatment her doctor has prescribed is the best way to go. I need a second doctor to agree that her case is being handled according to the latest available technology. I know a nationally recognized oncologist. I'm going to mail him a copy of her chart and ask him to read it so he can talk to me on the phone about her case. I trust his opinion and know he'll be honest with me because he doesn't know any of

Analysis

N: Another response that reflects the relative's concerns.

N: This response reflects the relative's decision to postpone any decision until after she meets with her mother's doctor.

N: This response asks the daughter to evaluate her final solution.

Interaction

the doctors in town. If he agrees with her present treatment and thinks everything possible is being done, I'll feel relieved. If he thinks something else could be done or there is cause for concern, I'll bring in a second doctor to see my mother.

N: You're going to discuss your mother's case with a doctor you know in another town. You're confident he will be perfectly honest and candid in giving you his opinion of her treatment.

R: I'm going to send her records to him by overnight delivery. Hopefully he'll be able to talk to me tomorrow afternoon. I did talk to him a couple of times before this, but he said it was really hard to make a judgment over the phone. He really needs to see my mother's chart before he can discuss the details of her treatment with me. I want to have talked with him before I see her doctor this week. That way, I'll already have the benefit of a second opinion.

N: Sounds like you're all set, and if you need to talk again, you know I'm available.

Analysis

N: This response reflects the daughter's evaluation of the final solution.

N: This response ends the interaction and invites the relative to recontact the nurse in the future.

SITUATION 5: DYING PATIENTS

Death is part of nursing. Nurses in oncology, intensive care, and infectious diseases routinely face death. They are often called on to comfort dying patients, discuss death, and help patients face their impending death with dignity. Listening to dying patients is a unique skill. The problems they present often have no solution. Besides basic listening/responding skills, listening to a dying patient requires a tremendous amount of patience and understanding. It is important not to minimize a patient's illness or to give a patient false hope. Most relatives are afraid to talk with their loved one about his or her impending death, but the patient still needs to talk and to voice fears, hopes, and concerns. It is important for the nurse to provide this role. Often there is no one else.

Dr. Elizabeth Kubler-Ross pioneered communication with dying patients. After extensive interviews with hundreds of dying patients, she defined five stages of dying: denial and isolation, anger, bargaining, depression, and acceptance. Understanding these stages, which are experienced universally by dying patients, is central to communicating effectively with them.

In order to understand better how to communicate with dying patients, the five stages of dying will be illustrated by using examples from AIDS patients and their families. Of all dying patients nurses must listen to, AIDS patients pose the ultimate challenge. AIDS is a long and painful disease, it poses a risk to the health community, it is often socially unacceptable, it is expensive, and the patient with AIDS often receives limited support from family and friends.

Parents.   Most gay AIDS patients have not told their parents of their sexual preference. Now that they are hospitalized, they not only have to tell their parents that they are gay but also that they have AIDS and they are going to die. Some parents react with love and acceptance, others are shocked, and many reject their sons, leaving them to die alone. Fathers have a harder time dealing with their son's homosexuality than mothers because fathers usually see it as a rejection of their masculinity.

Society.   AIDS patients generally keep their illness a secret from members of society because the reaction to the illness is so intense. Patients frequently tell stories about cab drivers who won't pick them up, doctors who hide them in the back room of the emergency room, dentists who refuse to treat them, and neighbors who pretend not to know them. The strong reaction of society toward AIDS patients increases the level of isolation experienced by AIDS patients and heightens their need to talk.

Employment. AIDS patients worry about losing their jobs. Often absent from work during the initial stages of their illness, they worry that their high level of absenteeism will result in termination. Forced to fabricate excuses for their absenteeism, they fear if their employer finds out they have AIDS, they will lose their job. AIDS patients also worry that they will have difficulty finding a job if they lose their current job. They believe no one will knowingly hire a person with AIDS.

Financial concerns. AIDS is an expensive disease. The medical costs incurred and the loss of income experienced result in serious financial concerns for all but the most affluent AIDS patients.

Insurance. AIDS patients worry that their insurance will be cancelled or that they are uninsurable. They also worry that they will reach the limits of their coverage, or that they will be unable to pay even their portion of the extensive medical bills they will incur.

AIDS itself. Most AIDS patients have generally read a lot about the disease and know someone who has died of AIDS. They know the course of the illness, the rapid rate in which it progresses, and the symptomology. They know that AIDS is a very painful disease and that before their death they will be disfigured and dependent. AIDS patients suffer from Kaposi's Sarcoma, colds, pneumonia, sores in the mouth, and weight loss. Knowing what lies ahead, many ask their friends and/or relatives to help them take their own lives.

When talking to AIDS patients, it is important to be aware of the five stages of dying, as well as the unique issues that confront AIDS patients.

Denial.   During denial, the first stage of dying, the patient denies he or she has a critical illness. A patient who fails to go to the hospital to get a blood test for the AIDS virus, even though symptoms of AIDS are being experienced, is exhibiting this stage of dying. Instead of getting a positive diagnosis, the person excuses the initial stages of illness as the flu. Families of a dying patient may also exhibit denial. A mother may deny her son's homosexuality and AIDS diagnosis. She may request a second or a third opinion, certain that the doctor or lab has made a mistake.

Anger.   Once an individual and his or her family accepts a critical diagnosis, anger usually follows. Statements like, "It's not fair," or "Why me?" typify the angry patient. Patients in this stage maybe angry at themselves or at others. An AIDS patient may be angry at himself or herself for ignoring safe-sex practices. Also, a lot of anger may be directed at the patient's lover for passing on the dreaded disease.

Bargaining.   During the third stage of dying, patients and their families try to bargain for more time. It is called bargaining rather than begging because with the request for more time is a promise to change. The form of a bargaining statement is, "God, if you let me live until ... then I promise ...." Promises are as unique as the patients themselves, but a few common promises are: "I'll never ask for anything again," "I'll give money to charity," "I'll become religious," or "I'll give up some sinful behavior." A woman with AIDS just wants to live to celebrate another Christmas. The parents of a young child with AIDS begs that their daughter might see the first day of school, hoping that by then medical science will have advanced enough to cure her.

Depression.   When critically ill patients accept their illness and their impending death as final, and realize there is no miracle cure and no way to bargain for additional time, depression results. Depression is particularly intense in AIDS patients and their families. Several factors unique to AIDS patients and their families contribute to this high level of depression. Because of the contagious nature of the disease, AIDS patients often do not get the emotional support from friends and relatives that other dying patients receive. Shame is also often associated with the disease because of how it was contracted. As a result, AIDS patients keep their illness a secret, resulting in an increased level of isolation and depression. Afraid to tell their friends and relatives what is wrong with their child for fear of public scorn or condemnation, families also experience an increased level of isolation.

AIDS patients also experience a heightened level of depression because they know the disease they have could have been avoided. Unlike cancer, which strikes without apparent warning or cause, the AIDS patient can generally say, "If I wouldn't have done this, then I wouldn't be in this situation." This high level of self-blame deepens the patient's level of depression.

Acceptance. Once a patient realizes that death is inevitable, and has been allowed to express anger and grief at the loss of his life, he or she can then accept the impending death peacefully. Dying patients, and more specifically AIDS patients, find peace in the last few hours, days, or weeks of life.

Talking to any dying patient requires extensive listening skills and sensitivity. Talking to an AIDS patient is no exception. The following dialogue is between a nurse and a hospitalized homosexual male patient with AIDS. The nurse concerned that the patient is depressed, initiates contact and invites the patient to talk. Read the dialogue carefully. See if you can identify the types of responses the nurse is using, as well as the stages of dying indicated by the patient.

Interaction	**Analysis**
N: How are you doing today?	*N:* Friendly contact.
P: Fine.	*P:* Noncommitted response.
N: You say fine, but you don't look very happy.	*N:* Confronts patient regarding conflict between what the patient says and how he looks. Usually it is counterproductive to confront the patient so early in the conversation.

Interaction	Analysis
P: Why should I be happy? I'm going to die soon, aren't I?	*P:* Patient is angry at confrontation. Responds sarcastically.
N: You get upset when you think you might die soon.	*N:* The nurse reflects the patient's upset.
P: When you're in this bed, all you can do is think or sleep. And since I can't sleep, I think.	*P:* The patient responds by being more open.
N: You think a lot while lying in bed.	*N:* The nurse reflects the patient's statement.
P: Yeah. I think about the past year. It's been hell. I think about what will happen next and how I got here in the first place.	
N: You think a lot about being sick this past year.	*N:* The nurse reflects the first part of the patient's statement, which results in the patient talking about his past year. If the nurse would have responded with either, "You think a lot about what would happen next," or "you think a lot about how you got in this situation," the patient's response would have been completely different. This is a key response that directs the rest of the conversation.

Interaction	Analysis
P: I go over it and over it. You know, it took a long time before I realized I had AIDS. First, I had sores in my mouth, then I had a cold that wouldn't go away. My body was unable to stop anything. I never really felt healthy. It was one thing after another	
N: When you first got sick, you didn't realize you had AIDS.	*N:* The nurse reflects the main point of the patient's statement.
P: No, I didn't. I knew something major was wrong with me. I thought possible it could be AIDS, but since the doctor I was seeing never mentioned AIDS, neither did I.	*P:* The patient admits he initially denied his illness.
N: You thought you could have AIDS, but you didn't want to face it.	*N:* The nurse reflects the denial, emphasizing the first stage of dying.
P: I thought it was likely since I've seen other people with AIDS, but I didn't think I could catch it. I don't know why I was so stupid.	
N: You didn't think you would catch AIDS.	*N:* The nurse reflects the patient's thoughts.

Interaction	Analysis
P: No, I didn't. I mean I knew all about the risks. What gay man doesn't? And who hasn't heard of safe sex? But I just thought if I used a rubber it would be an insult to my partner. I might as well have shouted, "I DON'T TRUST YOU."	*P:* The patient expands thoughts.
N: You knew you were taking a risk when you had sex unprotected.	*N:* Again, the nurse reflects thoughts.
P: Yeah, I knew. I guess I'm to blame for my own illness. When I first found out I did have AIDS, and I'll tell you it took a while, I had a sense of relief. At least now I knew what was wrong with me, I thought. I knew I was going to die, but it hadn't hit me yet.	
N: At first when you found out you had AIDS, you felt relieved. Now you feel differently.	*N:* The nurse reflects the patient's statement and prompts the patient for current feelings.
P: Now I feel so many things. For a while all I felt was anger, a raging anger. I would walk around the house and kick things. I was so angry I was	*P:* The patient expresses the second stage of dying — anger.

Interaction	**Analysis**
irrational. I was angry at everyone and every-thing.	
N: Who were you mad at?	*N:* The nurse questions for clarification of the statement, "everyone and everything."
P: I was angry at the government for not trying to find a cure for AIDS. They don't care because it's a gay disease. I was angry at my lover for giving me the disease. He should have told me he was HIV positive. But I guess I was most angry at myself, for being stupid, for taking unnecessary risks.	
N: But you're not angry now. What happened?	*N:* The nurse reflects current behavior, which is different from past behavior.
P I guess my anger just kind of burned itself out. You can only be that angry for so long and then you realize that it's doing no good. It's getting me nowhere.	
N: What happened next?	*N:* The nurse questions the patient regarding progress of events.

Interaction	Analysis
P: I tried to fight it. I read about different cures. I tried a high-vitamin diet. I wanted to buy more time. I tried every lead. But nothing worked.	*P:* The patient describes the bargaining stage.
N: You tried different cures in order to bargain for more time.	*N:* The nurse reflects the patient's bargaining.
P: Yeah. But none of them worked. I just kept getting worse. I guess I resigned myself to it. I'm going to die and I can't stop it.	
N: You feel there is nothing you can do to extend your life.	*N:* The nurse reflects the patient's feelings.
P: There isn't. It's futile. I guess that's why I'm so depressed. I feel helpless.... You know, it's hard watching someone else die but that's nothing compared to facing your own death. I'm scared. I never thought I would be. But I am. When you look death right in the eye, it's scary.	*P:* The patient begins a description of the fourth stage of dying.
N: You're depressed because you know you're going to die and you're not ready.	*N:* The patient expressed two feelings: fear and depression. The nurse decides to reflect depression, and the patient follows her lead.

Interaction	**Analysis**
P: No, I'm not ready. There is so much more I wanted to do. I wanted to travel — I've always wanted to go to China. And I wanted to see my sister's children grow up. I'm very close to them.	
N: You expected to live longer and do more with your life.	*N:* The nurse summarizes the patient's statement.
P: I would have, too, if I hadn't been so stupid. (Crying) Why was I so stupid? Why was I so stupid?	
N: You blame yourself for your illness.	*N:* The nurse clarifies the patient's statement.
P: Who else can I blame? I knew the risks. They just don't seem real. . . They just didn't seem real. Now it's all too real. All too scarey.	
N: Is there anything I can do to help, to make it less scarey?	*N:* The nurse offers support.
P: Not really. There's nothing anyone can do. I have to walk this last mile alone — I know that. I'm lucky I have the support of my family and friends. So many guys I know didn't have that. Their	

Interaction	**Analysis**
families disowned them and their lovers left them. They had to do all this alone.	
N: You have a lot of people who care about you.	N: The nurse reflects the positive.
P: I guess I should be grateful for that. It could be worse — a lot worse.	
N: I care about you, too. If you need anything, let me know.	N: The nurse again offers support.
P: I will. Hey — thanks for listening. It was a big help.	
N: Anytime.	
P: Thanks again.	

10
The Orchestration

Putting It

All Together

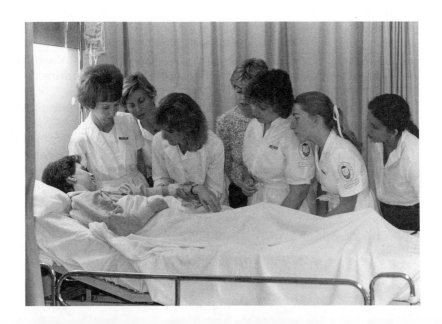

The integration of verbal and nonverbal behavior within a caring and authentic context is a challenging task for the professional helping person as well as for others. Understanding is communicated verbally through the content of the message. This content encompasses the person's cognitive and affective disclosures. Understanding is conveyed nonverbally by behavior that is congruent with the speaker's feelings. In a sense, verbal behavior within the facilitative relationship says "I understand what you're thinking and how you're feeling," and nonverbal behavior says "I'm with you and I'm feeling what you're feeling." When discrepancies between your verbal and your nonverbal behavior arise, it is wise to acknowledge and deal with them, since they are probably indicators of areas in your life that you have not resolved. Make the effort—stretch to understand your communications with others; it will be a growth-producing and enriching experience for you both as a person and as a professional.

Respect is communicated verbally by content that says "I value you as a person and I value your abilities and beliefs." Respect and caring are communicated nonverbally by behavior that is open and attentive and says "I have time to listen and to hear all that you wish to share with me. I am interested in you and in what you have to say." If you should ever find yourself uninterested in a patient or unable to value the other as a person, question the situation: perhaps the communication is not honest and your lack of interest is a response to the lack of genuineness.

If it's difficult for you to communicate respect for a particular person, ask yourself whether the cause is in the patient or in yourself. Again, struggle to understand your responses; they are helpful and provide valuable insights into yourself, which in turn strengthens your further communications with others.

Listening to and understanding patients on a personal level will prove to be an experience of growth for you as well as for your patients. They will come to know and understand themselves better, and you will come to know and understand yourself and others in the process. Whenever you are in doubt, be honest and genuine; share your thoughts and feelings with the patients: if you don't know what to say or how to respond, share that with the patient. Try to make the principles suggested in this manual your own. If you find yourself slipping, come back to the manual, read, and try the exercises again. Each time you read it, you should be able to improve your insight into and your understanding of your interactions with others. Above all, keep trying. Your patients need you.

11
Simulation Activities

Activity: Voice Analysis
Activity: Nonverbal Dyads
Activity: Communication of Emotion
Activity: Reflective-Interaction Triads
Activity: Extended Triad Interaction
Activity: Strengths and Weaknesses of
*   Reflection*
Activity: Understanding Others
Activity: Clarification-Interaction Triads
Activity: Extended Clarification Triad
*   Interaction*
Activity: Strengths and Weaknesses of
*   Clarification*
Activity: Response Practice
Activity: Interviewing
Activity: Beginning
Activity: Formulating Questions
Activity: Formulating Open Questions
Activity: Strengths and Weaknesses of
*   Questioning*
Activity: Response Analyses

ACTIVITY: VOICE ANALYSIS

Purpose

1. To give participants practice in listening for vocal clues.
2. To give participants feedback about how their voices sound to others.

Procedure

1. Participants pick a partner.
2. Partners sit back to back.
3. Both partners are to carry on a conversation with their eyes closed to cut off all other stimuli. Pay special attention not only to what the person is saying but also to how he or she is saying it. Listen to the tone of your partner's voice: Is it soothing, harsh, warm, excited?
4. The discussions should last for approximately 10 minutes.
5. Partners now face each other and give each other feedback on voice quality and tone.

Follow-up

1. What words would you use to describe your partner's voice?
2. Are what was said and how it was said in tune with each other or how are they contradictory?
3. If they were contradictory, which message did you believe, the verbal or the nonverbal one?

ACTIVITY: NONVERBAL DYADS

Purpose

1. To be aware of the nonverbal behavior of others.
2. To explore the meaning of nonverbal behavior.

Procedure

1. Participants should select a partner for this activity.
2. One person in each pair tells the other person about something significant that has happened to him or her recently.
3. The listener copies the nonverbal behavior of the speaker, acting as a mirror. He or she reflects the nonverbal behavior of the speaker.
4. After 5 minutes, the pair should discuss what happened.
5. The two should switch roles so that the listener becomes the speaker and the speaker becomes the listener.
6. The new listener mirrors the new speaker's nonverbal behavior.

Follow-up

1. What was the speaker's reaction to seeing his or her own nonverbal behavior?
2. How did the listener feel when he or she initiated the speaker's behavior?

ACTIVITY: COMMUNICATION OF EMOTION

Purpose

1. To acquaint participants with the various ways in which emotions and other states of being can be expressed nonverbally.

Procedure

1. Each participant in the group draws from a hat a slip of paper on which has been written an emotion or state of being.
2. Each participant must portray to the group, *nonverbally*, what is written on the paper.
3. The group then tries to guess what is being expressed. Suggested emotions and states of being are: anger, happiness, hatred, relaxation, depression, grief, tension, frustration, disappointment, disgust, confusion, worry, tiredness, nervousness, excitement, hesitancy, suspicion, discouragement, hostility, and joy.

Follow-up

1. What clues did you use in guessing what was being expressed—parts of the body, general posture, facial expression, type of body movement?
2. Was it hard to guess what was being expressed? If so, why?

ACTIVITY: REFLECTIVE-INTERACTION TRIADS

Purpose

1. To give participants practice in constructing reflective responses.
2. To give participants practice in discriminating between reflective and nonreflective responses.

Procedure

1. Participants break up into groups of three.
2. In each triad one participant is a speaker, one a listener, and one an observer.
3. The speaker takes one of the situations on the sentence completion sheet (p. 328) and completes the stem. When completing it, the speaker should provide the listener with more than a one-sentence stimulus. Completions that are three to five sentences in length work very well.
4. The listener then reflects the speaker's message.
5. The speaker next tells the listener whether the reflection was an accurate representation of the original message.
6. The role of the observer is, first, to determine whether the listener's response was a reflection (providing reasons for the decision), and, second, to analyze the focus of the reflection. Finally, the observer points to any other interesting aspects of the interaction.
7. Any other aspects of the interaction are discussed at this point.
8. This activity is repeated six times, with the participants each getting a chance to play each role twice.

Time	Speaker	Listener	Observer
1	A	B	C
2	B	A	C
3	A	C	B
4	C	A	B
5	B	C	A
6	C	B	A

A, B, and C are the three participants.

Follow-up

1. How difficult was it to keep making reflective responses?

Sentence-Completion Sheet

Situations

When I'm alone I...
When meeting new people, I...
At parties I...
Around the house I...
In strange places I...
At work I...
For fun I...
Being in school, I...
At night I...
When I don't know what to do, I...

Relationships

My mother....
My father...
My sister...
My brother...
My grandmother...
My grandfather...
My husband...
My wife...
A teacher of mine...
My boss...
My employees...
My best friend...
My boyfriend...
My girlfriend...
A friend of mine...

ACTIVITY: EXTENDED TRIAD INTERACTION

Purpose

1. To provide practice in making reflective responses.
2. To provide practice in discriminating between reflective and nonreflective responses.
3. To provide an opportunity to experience and observe what happens when the reflective response is continuously implemented.
4. To provide an opportunity to experience how the speaker responds to a reflective response.

Procedure

1. Participants break up into groups of three.
2. In each triad one participant is a speaker, one a listener, and one an observer.
3. The speaker thinks of a problem that he or she will feel comfortable talking about for 10 minutes. The problem and its ramifications should be clear in the speaker's mind before the discussion begins.
4. The speaker discusses the problem. The listener responds to the speaker by using *only* the reflective response. The interaction should last from 5 to 10 minutes.
5. At the completion of the interaction, all three participants should discuss what occurred in the interaction. In this discussion, each participant should contribute his or her unique experience of what occurred. The listener should relay the thoughts and feelings he or she had during the interaction, as well as the difficulties, if any, of attempting to use only the reflective response. The speaker should relay how he or she felt during the interaction and what his or her reaction was to the listener. The observer should be able to point out deviations from the reflective response style and give an objective view of the total interaction.
6. The activity is repeated three times. Each participant is to play each role once.

Time	Speaker	Listener	Observer
1	A	B	C
2	C	A	B
3	B	C	A

A, B, and C are the three participants.

Follow-up

1. How difficult was it to keep making only reflective responses?
2. What problems arose during the interaction?
3. What caused the interaction to end?
4. How did the reflective response affect the speaker's behavior?

ACTIVITY: STRENGTHS AND WEAKNESSES OF REFLECTION

Purpose

1. To examine the strengths and weaknesses of the reflective response.

Procedure

1. Participants break up into groups of four to six.
2. Each group appoints a secretary.
3. Each group discusses the strengths and weaknesses of the reflective response.
4. When the group agrees on a strength or a weakness, the secretary writes it down.
5. Each group tries to record as many strengths and weaknesses as possible in the time allotted. (A reasonable time limit is 15 minutes.)
6. Each group then presents its results to the entire group of participants.

ACTIVITY: UNDERSTANDING OTHERS

Purpose

1. To give participants practice in imagining how another person might think and feel about a situation.

Procedure

1. Each participant in the group thinks of a problem situation that he or she has faced that was particularly emotional.
2. Each person then describes the situation in writing, being careful not to include any thoughts or feelings about the situation. No name or other identifying marks should be on the paper.
3. All written situations are put in a paper bag.
4. Each participant then draws a paper from the bag and reads the situation to the group. The person then tells the group how he or she believes the person who described the situation thought and felt about that situation.

Follow-up

1. If the person whose paper was read wishes to do so, he or she may indicate whether the reader's interpretation of the thoughts and feelings involved was correct.
2. Participants who are listening to the reader's opinion of the thoughts and feelings involved also may offer their own opinions on the subject.

ACTIVITY: CLARIFICATION-INTERACTION TRIADS

Purpose

1. To give participants practice in making reflective responses.
2. To give participants practice in discriminating between reflective and nonreflective responses.

Procedure

1. Participants break up into groups of three.
2. In each triad, one person is the speaker, one is the listener, and one is the observer.
3. The speaker chooses one of the situations on the sentence-completion sheet (p. 334) and completes the stem. In completing it, the speaker should use at least three or four sentences and they should be true representations of his or her feelings.
4. The listener elaborates (clarifies) the speaker's message.
5. The speaker then tells the listener whether the elaboration was an accurate representation of his or her feelings and, if it was not accurate, exactly what the listener misunderstood.
6. The role of the observer is to determine whether the speaker's response was a clarification and to give reasons for that decision. The observer should also analyze the focus of the listener's response: Does the response focus on the listener's thoughts and feelings, or the thoughts and feelings of the speaker? The observer should also point out any other interesting aspects of the interaction.
7. All members of the triad may discuss any other aspects of the interaction at this point.
8. This activity is repeated six times. Each participant will have two chances to be the speaker, to be the listener, and to be the observer.

Time	Speaker	Listener	Observer
1	A	B	C
2	B	A	C
3	A	C	B
4	C	A	B
5	B	C	A
6	C	B	A

A, B, and C are the three participants.

Sentence-Completion Sheet

Feelings

I feel especially happy when...
The time I felt most embarrassed was when I...
What frustrates me the most is...
It makes me angry when...
It makes me sad to think about...
I had the time of my life when...
I really enjoy...
I never felt so low as when...
It is very hard for me to think about...
I hesitate whenever...
It's important for me to...
I cry when I think about...

ACTIVITY: EXTENDED CLARIFICATION TRIAD INTERACTION

Purpose

1. To provide practice in making clarification responses.
2. To provide practice in discriminating between clarifying and nonclarifying responses.
3. To provide an opportunity to experience and observe what happens when the clarification response is continuously implemented.
4. To provide an opportunity to experience how a speaker responds to a clarification response.

Procedure

1. Participants break up into groups of three.
2. In each triad one participant is a speaker, one is a listener, and one an observer.
3. The speaker thinks of a problem that he or she will feel comfortable talking about for 10 minutes. The problem and its ramifications should be clear in the speaker's mind before the discussion begins.
4. The speaker discusses the problem. The listener responds by using *only* clarification responses. The interaction should last from 5 to 10 minutes.
5. At the end of the interaction, all three participants should discuss the process of the interaction. In this discussion, each participant should contribute his or her unique experience of what occurred. The listener should relay the thoughts and feelings he or she had during the interaction and the difficulties he or she had, if any, in attempting to use only clarification responses. The speaker should also tell what his or her reaction was to the listener. The observer should be able to point out deviations from the clarification response style and give a more objective view of the total interaction.
6. The activity is repeated three times. Each participant is to play each role once.

Time	Speaker	Listener	Observer
1	A	B	C
2	C	A	B
3	B	C	A

A, B, and C are the three participants.

Follow-up

1. How difficult was it to keep making clarification responses?
2. What problems arose during the interaction?
3. What caused the interaction to end?
4. How did the repeated use of clarification response affect the speaker's behavior?

ACTIVITY: STRENGTHS AND WEAKNESSES OF CLARIFICATION

Purpose

1. To examine the strengths and weaknesses of the clarification response.

Procedure

1. Participants break up into groups of four to six.
2. Each group appoints a secretary.
3. Each group discusses the strengths and weaknesses of the clarification response.
4. When the group agrees on a strength or a weakness, the secretary writes it down.
5. Each group tries to record as many strengths and weaknesses as possible in the time allotted. (A reasonable time limit is 15 minutes.)
6. Each group then presents its results to the entire group of participants.

ACTIVITY: RESPONSE PRACTICE

Purpose

1. To give students practice in responding with reflective and clarifying statements.
2. To give members of the group an opportunity to learn more about each other.

Procedure

1. Break up into groups of five to six.
2. Each participant receives seven 3X5 cards.
3. On each card, participants complete the following sentence:

I am a _____.

Possible responses might be:

I am a happy person.

I am a mother.

I am a teacher.

I am a horseback rider.

All sentence completions should provide accurate information about the participant.

4. This is a values activity, and it involves "giving up" the characteristics written on the cards. The participants pretend that they can no longer be whatever is written on the card. They are giving up that part of their identity.
5. Each member of the group, in turn, gives up one card and explains why that particular card is chosen. He or she should say something like "I'm going to give up (the card that was selected) because (reason for choosing that card)."

An example would be: "I'm going to give up being a teacher, since, although I enjoy working with kids, I can earn a living as a secretary. I've done that before, and I enjoyed it. I could interact with students as a volunteer."

6. The person to the right of the speaker reflects the speaker's statements and receives feedback from the entire group as to the accuracy of the reflections.
7. After all group members have given up one card, the process is repeated, each participant giving up a second card.
8. The process is repeated again.
9. After each participant has given up three cards, the activity is again repeated—but this time with a modification. The person to the right of the speaker *clarifies* the speaker's statement and receives feedback from the *speaker* about the accuracy of the clarification. This modification is repeated three times, at which point each participant should have one card left.
10. Each participant reads his or her last card to the rest of the group.
11. Free comments are then allowed on which card each person kept until last.

Follow-up

1. How difficult was it to "give up" parts of your identity?
2. Were other group members generally accurate in the their responses?
3. Did you learn anything about yourself?

ACTIVITY: INTERVIEWING

Purpose:

1. To explore the dynamics of questioning.
2. To examine the role of questions in obtaining information.

Procedure

1. Break into dyads.
2. One member of the pair interviews his or her partner. The purpose of the interview is to obtain as much information about the person as possible. During the exchange, the interviewer must exclusively ask questions. After five minutes, the interview is stopped.
3. Participants switch roles. This interview is also stopped after five minutes.
4. Dyads will discuss the interview process. They should consider how much information was received and how the interviewee felt about the interview process.
5. Dyads will now interview each other again. This time, the participants will try to obtain as much information about his or her partner without asking any questions at all. Each interview will again last a total of five minutes.
6. Partners will now discuss the interaction again.

Follow-up

1. How did you respond when you were being asked a long list of questions? How did you feel?
2. How did you respond when no questions were being presented to you? How did you feel?
3. Compare your reactions to the two situations. Which was more successful?
4. What types of questions did you ask?
5. Which were the most successful in obtaining information?

ACTIVITY: BEGINNING

Purpose

1. To develop a set of alternatives for beginning an interview.
2. To learn how to analyze the effectiveness of opening questions.

Procedure

1. Break into groups of four to six participants.
2. Each group should appoint a recorder to takes notes during the rest of the session.
3. The members of each group now brainstorm questions and statements that can be used to initiate interactions with a patient.
4. After all possible suggestions are recorded, evaluate each suggestion. Members of the group should discuss each of the suggested alternatives, paying particular attention to the level of interest and the respect communicated.
5. After each of the suggested opening statements is evaluated, the group should "star" the two best alternatives.
6. Each group of participants should write its two best opening statements on the blackboard.

Follow-up

1. Is there any similarity to the opening statements selected?
2. Are there any other characteristics that they all seem to have?
3. Are there any other qualities that you think are critical to a good opening statement?
4. How important do you think the nurse's initial statement is to the entire interaction process?

ACTIVITY: FORMULATING QUESTIONS

Purpose

1. To practice formulating different types of questions.
2. To analyze different types of questions.

Procedure

1. Break into groups of four to six participants.
2. Provide each group with a copy of the stimulus statements.
3. One member of the group reads Stimulus Statement A to the rest of the group.
4. Group members brainstorm a series of questions they would ask Client A in response to the stimulus statement as if they were the counselor. A recorder, appointed by the groups, records all suggestions.
5. Each question suggested is evaluated in terms of the amount of empathic understanding and respect it communicates. Suggestions should be made on how to increase the empathic understanding and respect communicated by the questions.
6. The procedure is repeated for Stimulus Statement B.

Follow-up

1. How effective are questions in communicating empathy and respect?
2. What types of questions have a higher empathic communication than others?
3. How effective were you in communicating empathy and respect in the form of questions?

Stimulus Statements for Formulating Questions

Stimulus Statement A

I don't have any energy. I can't seem to do anything. It's such a struggle just to get out of bed. All I want to do is sleep. I think my doctor is getting mad at me for not trying harder, but I don't even care. I've never felt this way before.

Stimulus Statement B

My family's disowned me just because I'm friends with Jim. Now is the time I really need their support and they are letting us down. I don't know how to approach them.

ACTIVITY: FORMULATING OPEN QUESTIONS

Purpose

1. To provide practice in formulating open questions.
2. To provide practice in changing closed questions into open questions.

Procedure

1. Break into groups of four to six.
2. Give each participant a copy of the stimulus statements with closed questions.
3. Each group will discuss the closed questions provided and reformulate them into open questions.
4. After the format of all closed questions has been changed, participants will read the questions and evaluate their significance to the client.
5. Additional significant open questions can be added to the list.

Follow-up

1. How difficult was it to reformulate closed questions into open questions?
2. How did reformulating the questions increase their significance to the patient?
3. How can you remind yourself to evaluate the significance of a question before asking it?

Stimulus Statement with Closed Questions

Stimulus Statement A

I don't know what to do. I'm afraid of people—afraid of getting too close to them. I mean I like people, I just don't know what to do. I think I like them too much. I start to get to know someone and it's okay. Then I fall head over heals for them. It scares me. I always end up getting hurt. That's how it happened with Jim.

Closed Questions

1. How many times did this happen before?
2. Would you say you were in love with Jim?
3. You'd like me to tell you what to do?

4. Are you afraid of people hurting you or you hurting people?
5. Was Jim in love with you?

Stimulus Statement B

I don't know what to do. My husband's going to be mining out in the desert all summer. He wants me to go out there and spend the summer with him. What if I get sick? I'm kind of scared. I'm a diabetic. Plus, if I stay here I can work and earn some extra money, but then I might not see my husband for months!

Closed Question

1. Where is your husband mining?
2. How long will he be gone?
3. What are you afraid of?
4. How much money do you make at work?
5. How much money is your husband earning mining?
6. Is your diabetes serious?

ACTIVITY: STRENGTHS AND WEAKNESSES OF QUESTIONING

Purpose

1. To examine the strengths and weaknesses of questioning.

Procedure

1. Participants break into groups of four to six.
2. Each group appoints a secretary.
3. Each group discusses the strengths and weaknesses of the clarification response.
4. When the group agrees on a strength or a weakness, the secretary writes it down.
5. Each group tries to record as many strengths and weaknesses as possible in the time allotted. (A reasonable time limit is 15 minutes.)
6. Each group then presents its results to the entire group of participants.

ACTIVITY: RESPONSE ANALYSES

Purpose

1. To encourage participants to analyze how they interact with people they know.

Procedure

1. Using a tape recorder, record an interaction (lasting 15 to 30 minutes) with someone you know fairly well. Try to behave as you usually do with this person.
2. After recording the interaction, listen to the tape and classify your statements as reflection, questioning, clarification, or other.
3. How did your voice sound? Analyze the pitch, the tone, and your choice of words.

Follow-up

1. How many responses of each type did you make?
2. What was your predominant style?
3. What is your reaction to your interaction style?
4. Would you like to change any aspects of the way you behaved? If so, which aspects?

References

Allport, G. 1955. *Becoming*. New Haven: Yale University Press.

Barbara, D. A. 1974. *The art of listening*. Springfield, IL: Charles C. Thomas.

Barelson, B., & Steiner, G. 1964. *Human behavior*. New York: Harcourt, Brace & World.

Berenson, B. G., & Carkhuff, R. R. (Eds.) 1967. *Sources of gain in counseling and psychotherapy*. New York: Holt, Rinehart & Winston.

Bernstein, L., Bernstein, R. S., & Dana, R., II. 1985. *Interviewing: A guide for health professionals* (4th ed.). New York: Appleton and Lange.

Bugental, J. F. T. (Ed.). 1967. *Challenges of humanistic psychology*. New York: Macmillan.

Burnard, P. 1985. "Learning to communicate." *Nursing Mirror* 8:30-31.

_____. 1987. "Meaningful dialogue." *Nursing Times* 20:34-45.

Carkhuff, R. R. 1987. *The art of helping* (6th ed.). Amherst, MA: Human Resources Development Press.

_____, & Berenson, B. G. 1967. *Beyond counseling and psychotherapy*. New York: Holt, Rinehart & Winston.

_____. 1969. *Helping and human relations: A primer for lay and professional helpers*. New York: Holt, Rinehart & Winston.

_____. 1985. *Productive problem solving*. Amherst, MA: Human Resources Development Press.

Carlson, C. E. (Ed.). 1970. *Behavioral concepts and nursing intervention*. Philadelphia: Lippincott.

Carson, R. C. 1970. *Interaction concepts of personality*. Chicago: Aldine.

Combs, A. W., Richards, A. C., & Richards, F. 1976. *Perceptual psychology: A humanistic approach to the study of persons*. New York: Harper & Row.

Corey, G. 1985. *A case approach to counseling and psychotherapy* (2nd ed.). Monterey, CA: Brooks/Cole.

_____. 1985. *Theory and practice of counseling and psychotherapy* (3rd ed.). Monterey, CA: Brooks/Cole.

Culbert, S. A. 1970. *The interpersonal process of self-disclosure: It takes two to see one.* Fairfax, VA: Human Resources, NTL.

Cushnie, P. 1988. "Conflict: Developing resolution skills." *AORN Journal* 3:732, 734-45.

Egan, G. 1973. *Face to face.* Monterey, CA: Brooks/Cole.

_____. 1985. *The skilled helper: Model skills and methods for effective helping* (3rd ed.). Monterey, CA: Brooks/Cole.

_____. 1976. *Interpersonal living: A skills/contract approach to human relations training in groups.* Monterey, CA: Brooks/ Cole.

Evans, K., & Hind, T. 1987. "Getting the message across." *Nursing Times* 18:40-42.

Faulkner, A. 1986. "Human interest." *Nursing Times* 20:43-45.

Gazda, G. M., Walters, R. P., & Childers, W. C. 1975. *Human relations development: A manual for health sciences.* Boston: Allyn and Bacon.

_____. 1982. *Interpersonal communication: A handbook for health professionals.* Rockville, MD: Aspen.

Gobel, F. 1984. *A third force: The psychology of Abraham Maslow.* New York: Grossman.

Hannah, G. 1987. "Getting your wires crossed." *Nursing Times* 41:64-65.

Henrick, A. P. 1984. "What's really bothering your patient? 5 ways to find out." *Nursing Life* 5:62-64.

Hein, E. C. 1980. *Communication in nursing practice* (2nd ed.). Boston: Little, Brown.

Jacobs, K., Jonathan, B., McCollin, A., & Wells, D. 1986. "Facilitating the nurse's role as a communicator: The design and use of a communication record." *Perspectives* 3:7-9.

Jourard, S. M. 1970. *Disclosing man to himself.* New York: Van Nostrand Reinhold.

_____. 1971. *The transparent self* (Rev. ed.). New York: Van Nostrand Reinhold.

_____. 1980. *Healthy personality: An approach from the viewpoint of humanistic psychology* (4th ed.). New York: Macmillan.

Kalisch, B. 1971. "An experiment in the development of empathy in nursing students." *Nursing Research* 20:202-11.

Kasch, C. 1984. "Interpersonal competence and communication in the delivery of nursing care." *Advances in Nursing Science* 2:71-78.

_____. 1986. "Toward a theory of nursing action: Skills and competency in nurse-patient interaction." *Nursing Research* 4:226-30.

King, I. M. 1981. *A theory for nursing systems: Systems, concepts, and process.* New York: Wiley.

Kratochvil, D. 1969. "Changes in values and in interpersonal functioning of nurses in training." *Counselor Education and Supervision* 8:104-07.

Kron, T. 1972. *Communication in nursing.* Philadelphia: Saunders.

Kubler-Ross, E. 1987. *AIDs: The ultimate challenge.* New York: Macmillan.

Lewis, G. K. 1978. *Nurse-patient communication* (3rd ed.). Dubuque, IA: Brown.

Mayeroff, M. 1972. *On caring.* New York: Harper & Row.

McAlvanah, M. 1988. "Communication: A two way street." *Pediatric Nursing* 2:140-60.

Montagu, A. 1971. *Touching: The human significance of the skin.* New York: Columbia University Press.

Orem, D. E. 1985. *Nursing: Concepts of practice* (3rd ed.). New York: McGraw-Hill.

Orlando, I. J. 1972. *The discipline and teaching of nursing process.* New York: Putnam's.

Otto, H. A., & Knight, J. W. (Eds.) 1979. *Dimensions in wholestic healing: New frontiers in the treatment of the whole person.* Chicago: Nelson Hall.

_____, & Mann, J. 1968. *Ways of growth.* New York: Viking Press.

Patterson, C. H. 1985. *Theories of counseling and psychotherapy* (4th ed.). New York: Harper & Row.

Peplau, H. E. 1952. *Interpersonal relations in nursing.* New York: Putnam's.

Pinel, C. 1984. "Say what you mean." *Nursing Mirror* 24:22-23.

Quinn, M. 1986. "Whose turn is it to break the silence?" *Nursing Times* 42:47-48.

Rogers, C. R. 1972. *On becoming a person.* Boston: Houghton Mifflin.

_____. 1965. *Client-centered therapy.* Boston: Houghton Mifflin.

_____. 1983. *Freedom to learn for the eighties.* Columbus, OH: Merrill.

Rogers, M. E. 1970. *An introduction to the theoretical basis of nursing.* Philadelphia: F. A. Davis.

Roy, C. 1984. *Introduction to nursing: An adaptation model* (2nd ed.). Englewood Cliffs, NJ: Prentice-Hall.

Travelbee, J. 1966. *Interpersonal aspects of nursing.* Philadelphia: F. A. Davis.

Truax, C. B., & Wargo, D. G. 1966. "Psychotherapeutic encounters that change behavior: For better or for worse." *American Journal of Psychotherapy* 22: 499-520.

_____, & Carkhuff, R. R. 1967. *Toward effective counseling and psychotherapy: Training and practice.* Chicago: Aldine.

Tubbs, S. L., & Moss, S. 1983. *Human communication: An interpersonal perspective.* New York: Random House.

Van Kaam, A. 1984. *Existential foundation of psychology.* New York: University Press of America.

Watson, D L., & Tharp, R. G. 1988. *Self-directed behavior: Self-modification for personal adjustment* (5th ed.). Monterey, CA: Brooks/Cole.

Weigert, E. 1970. *The courage to be and to love.* New Haven, CN: Yale University Press.

Yura, H., & Walsh, M. B. 1987. *The nursing press: Assessing, planning, implementing, evaluating.* New York: Appleton and Lange.

_____. 1978. *Human needs and the nursing process.* New York: Appleton-Century-Crofts.

Index